SECRETS TO COMMUNICATING WITH YOUR CHILD WITH AUTISM

YOUR CHILD IS TRYING TO COMMUNICATE WITH YOU. HERE'S HOW YOU CAN UNDERSTAND THEM.

MARIA ELENA REYES-SCHAFER, M.S., M.ED.

JAMES C. SCHAFER, MBA $

CONTENTS

DISCLAIMER

This book is designed to provide information on the topic of Autism Spectrum Disorder culture only. This information is provided and sold with the knowledge that the publisher and authors do not offer any legal or medical advice. In case of a need for any such expertise, consult with the appropriate professional. This book does not contain all information available on the subject. This book has not been created to be specific to any individual person or organization's situation or needs. Reasonable efforts have been made to make this book as accurate as possible. However, there may be typographical and or content errors. Therefore, this book should serve only as a general guide. This book contains information that might be dated or erroneous and is intended only to educate and entertain. The authors and publisher shall have no liability or responsibility to any person or entity regarding any loss or damage incurred, or alleged to have incurred, directly or indirectly, by the information contained in this book or as a result of anyone acting or failing to act upon the information in this book. You hereby agree to be bound by this disclaimer, covenant not to sue and release. You may return this book within the guaranteed time period for a full refund. In the interest of full disclosure, this book may contain affiliate links that might pay the author or publisher a commission upon any purchase from the company. While the authors and publisher take no responsibility for any virus or technical issues that could be caused by such links, the business practices of these companies, and or the performance of any

DEDICATION

Every child is unique in their own way, and I'd like to dedicate this book to the thousands of children with special needs that I have had the distinct privilege of working with to develop a sense of connection and trust and to the many more whom I will meet in the future through our ASD Parent Network. No amount of academic training can compare to the lessons and wisdom that I have gained from these precious children and time spent with them. I would also like to acknowledge the support that I received from parents, colleagues, therapists, advocates, the community at large, as well as the subject matter experts, without whom this book would not have been possible. I would also like to thank my husband, who helped me make this book a reality and while not a subject matter expert in this field, has helped me transfer my expertise to a work that is meant to help families with communicating with their child with Autism. Finally, a special dedication must be made to a couple who I have had the privilege of working with for many years. You have shown an unwavering dedication to your children. You continue to trust in the community services and support systems that are available for children with special needs. These are the services that I discuss in this book which can improve the communication and social skills with children with autism.

Maria Elena Reyes Schafer, M. S., M. Ed.

ASDParentNetwork.com

Please visit our website https://ASDParentNetwork.com to receive free e-books on related topics as they are developed from the feedback we receive from this edition Secrets to Communicating With Your Child With Autism.

INTRODUCTION

You feel tired, frustrated, and dejected because no matter how hard you try, you can't seem to get through to your child on the spectrum, and they just can't seem to get their feelings across to you. All parents of children with autism have been there. The experience is completely normal, and it's only natural to seek help.

It goes without saying that communication between parent and child is crucial to early development, but communication is something that parents of neurotypical children take for granted. Children with Autism Spectrum Disorder, or ASD, generally experience difficulty expressing their thoughts and feelings, frustrating not only themselves but their parents as well. Of course, the blame cannot be placed on your child - they didn't ask to be born with ASD - nor can you blame yourself, because after all, no parent expects their child to be born with autism, and thus no parent is prepared for the challenges that a child on the spectrum may face and present.

There is perhaps nothing more heartbreaking than finding your child in tears, asking "Hey, what's wrong?" in that cooing voice that only a parent can achieve, and persist with the question, only to have your little one cry harder and louder. What could you do in this situation? Your child has no way of telling you what the problem might be, and you have no way of calming them down, telling them it's going to be okay.

Because of this lack of communication, a disconnect forms, and parent and child fail to bond.

Learning how to communicate meaningfully with your child with autism will bridge this gap and allow you to experience the full joys of parenthood without the frustration that you faced previously. You'll no longer have to struggle for hours trying to understand your child, or calm them down, or help them engage in healthy activities and interests. All of these things will become second nature, and soon enough, you and your child will be happier than ever.

With this book, you'll learn how to recognize certain behaviors that ASD children display, what they mean, and how you can respond to them in a positive, healthy way. You will learn various methods of communication and how to encourage healthy behaviors, and eventually, you'll become closer to your child than you could have possibly imagined.

Our passion for teaching parents of children on the spectrum how to achieve meaningful communication comes from a desire to see that all children on the spectrum receive the same level of comfort and care that non-ASD children do, despite the difficulties and frustrations that they may face. I've been helping parents of children with ASD, and indeed children with ASD themselves, for years, and have conducted extensive research to provide you with solutions for all autism-related problems in communication that you may have so that you can give your child the happiness they deserve, and the happiness you deserve as well.

Having the ability to communicate effectively with your child on the spectrum is the first step in providing them with the childhood they deserve. Are you ready to learn?

1

WHAT IS AUTISM SPECTRUM DISORDER?

If you've only recently learned that your child has Autism Spectrum Disorder, then you may not know precisely what that term means. Autism Spectrum Disorder, often shortened to ASD (which we'll do from this point forward), is a developmental and neurological disorder that begins in the early stages of childhood and lasts throughout the diagnosed individual's life. It affects how a person acts and interacts with others, learns, and of course, communicates. ASD includes what was known as Asperger syndrome and pervasive developmental disorder.

We called ASD a 'spectrum' disorder because people with autism can display a wide range of symptoms and behaviors. People with ASD may experience difficulty when trying to communicate with others or be averted to looking you in the eye when talking to others. Their interests may also be restricted, and they may display repetitive behaviors. ASD individuals might spend plenty of time organizing certain things or repeating the same phrase or sentence continuously. Autistic people, especially children, are often described as living in their own world.

At well-child checkups, your health care provider should monitor the development of your child. If your child displays signs of ASD, they will receive a comprehensive evaluation, which could include a team of specialists conducting a series of tests and evaluations to ensure an accurate diagnosis. We still don't know what causes ASD, but research strongly suggests that both environment and genes play important roles. There is currently no single standard treatment for ASD, though there are plenty of ways to improve your child's ability to learn new skills and grow. Starting early will often yield better results, and treatments include communication and behavior therapists, medicines to control symptoms, and skills training.

Let's take a closer look at the ins and outs of Autism Spectrum Disorder throughout this chapter.

A BRIEF EXPLANATION OF ASD

Like I mentioned previously, Autism Spectrum disorder is a developmental disorder that can cause significant communication, social, and behavioral challenges in the affected individual. There is generally nothing about the way that people with ASD look that differentiates them from non-ASD individuals. Still, people with ASD may interact, communicate, learn, and behave in ways that are atypical of people without autism. The thinking, learning, and problem-solving abilities of people with ASD can range from highly gifted to severely challenged. Some people with autism require a lot of assistance in their day to day lives, while others need barely any help at all.

An ASD diagnosis now includes several conditions that were previously diagnosed separately. They are autistic disorder, pervasive developmental disorder not otherwise specified (PDD-NOS), and Asperger syndrome. All of these conditions now fall under the umbrella term of Autism Spectrum Disorder.

The concept of a 'spectrum' autism diagnosis was created in the DSM-5, combining the previous edition's separate pervasive developmental disorder diagnoses into one. Rett syndrome is no longer included under the DSM-5's definition of ASD, as it is now considered its own neurological disorder. A separate social pragmatic communication disorder, or SPCD, was created for individuals with disabilities in social communication, but lacking restricted, repetitive behaviors. Moreover, severity level descriptors were included to aid in categorizing the level of support needed by an ASD individual.

This new definition was created to be more accurate and aims to help diagnose ASD earlier in an individual's life. However, studies calculating the potential impact of transitioning from the DSM-4 to the DSM- have predicted a decrease in the prevalence of ASD. There has been even more concern that children who were previously diagnosed with PDD-NOS would not meet the criteria for an ASD diagnosis.

As you can see, diagnosing ASD is not an easy task. Therefore, you must take your child to a trusted doctor for evaluation to avoid receiving an inaccurate diagnosis that may compromise your young one's health and well-being.

DIAGNOSING AUTISM

Doctors and medical professionals diagnose ASD by observing an individual's development and behavior. ASD can generally be diagnosed reliably by the age of two, and it is vital for parents with concerns to seek out assessment as soon as possible so that a diagnosis may be made and treatment and therapy can begin. The process of diagnosis in children is generally a two-stage process.

Stage 1 involves general developmental screening during well-child checkups. Every child should be receiving well-child checkups with an early childhood health care provider or a pediatrician. The American Academy of Pediatrics recommends that every child be screened for delays in development at their 9, 18, 24, or 30-month well-child checkups. Additional screening may be required if a child is at high risk for developmental problems like ASD. Those that are high-risk include children that have family members with ASD, have older parents, display some ASD behaviors, were born with very low birth weight, or have certain genetic conditions.

Your concerns and experiences as a parent are critical in your child's screening process, especially at a young age. A doctor will sometimes ask you questions regarding your child's behaviors and check those answers against information from screening tools for ASD, as well as with their observations of your child. Children that display developmental problems during this stage will be referred for the second evaluation stage.

The second evaluation involves a team of health professionals and doctors that have experience with diagnosing ASD. This team could include a child psychiatrist or psychologist that has specialized training in behavior and brain development, a developmental pediatrician that has training in child development, a speech-language pathologist that has had training in communication difficulties, and a neuropsychologist that focuses on assessing, diagnosing, and treating medical, neurological, and neurodevelopmental disorders. This evaluation might assess your child's language abilities, cognitive level (or thinking skills), and skills appropriate to their age needed for the independent performance of daily activities, like eating, toileting, and dressing.

Since ASD is a complex disorder that may sometimes accompany other learning disorders or illnesses, more comprehensive evaluations could include blood tests and hearing tests. The outcome of the evaluation will result in a formal, final diagnosis and recommendations for treatments. ASD symptoms that occur in older children and adolescents in school will often be recognized first by parents and teachers and then evaluated by the school's special education team. This team may perform an initial evaluation and recommend that these children visit specific doctors specializing in ASD for formal, traditional assessment.

Parents can talk with these specialists about the social difficulties that their child faces, including problems with nuanced, subtle communication. These subtle communication issues can include challenges in understanding facial expressions, tone of voice, or body language. Older children or adolescents can experience problems understanding humor, figures of speech, and sarcasm. Parents may also notice that their child has difficulty forming and building friendships with their peers.

Diagnosing autism in adults is generally more difficult than doing so in children. As adults, some symptoms of ASD can overlap with symptoms of other mental health disorders, like ADHD and anxiety. Adults that notice the symptoms and signs of ASD should speak to their doctor and request a referral for an evaluation. While the testing process for ASD in adults is still being refined, adults can be referred to a psychologist, neuropsychologist, or psychiatrist that has experience with ASD. These experts will ask about concerns with sensory issues, social interactions, communication challenges, restricted interests, and repetitive behaviors.

Information regarding the adult's developmental history will help the medical professional make an accurate diagnosis, so an ASD evaluation could include talking to parents or other family members. Receiving an accurate ASD diagnosis as an adult can help a person understand specific difficulties they may have faced in the past, obtain the right kind of help, and identify their strengths. There are currently studies being performed to determine the types of support and services most helpful for improving the community integration and functioning of transition-age youth and adults with Autism Spectrum Disorder.

THE TELLTALE SIGNS OF AUTISM SPECTRUM DISORDER

People with Autism Spectrum Disorder generally experience difficulty with social interaction and communication, repetitive behaviors, and restricted interest. While I'll be discussing some of the most common symptoms that people diagnosed with ASD display, not all people with autism will display all behaviors, but most will exhibit several.

One of the most common social behaviors that people with ASD display is the inability to make prolonged eye contact and make consistent eye contact. An individual with ASD may be resistant to making eye contact, and your attempts to make eye contact with them, which non-ASD individuals often misinterpret as a lack of interest in the conversation. Moreover, autistic individuals may tend not to look or listen to people, which once again mistakenly conveys the message that they are not interested in a conversation, leading to frustration on both ends.

Children with ASD will rarely express their enjoyment of activities or objects by showing things to others or pointing them out. They may also fail to or be slow to respond to someone calling their name or other verbal attempts at gaining their attention. This should once again not be interpreted as rude behavior. ASD children can display difficulty with the back and forth of conversation, often failing to respond to questions or statements made in a conversation.

The social issues that people with ASD face are not just common 'difficulties' like shyness, and they can cause significant problems in everyday life. Neurotypical children will be very interested in the people and world around them. By their first birthday, a toddler will generally interact with people by looking them in the eye, using simple gestures like waving or clapping, and copying words and actions. Non-ASD toddlers will also display interests in games, but young children with ASD may have difficulty learning to interact with others. Some children with ASD may not be interested in other people, while others might want friends but not understand how to develop and foster friendship. You may have noticed that your ASD child has difficulty learning how to share and take turns, far more than non-ASD children, which could make other children not want to play or interact with them.

One of the most difficult challenges that ASD children and parents of ASD children face is problems sharing or talking about their feelings. Children with autism might also experience difficulty understanding others' feelings, and many people with ASD are sensitive to touch and may not want to be cuddled or held. Self-stimulatory behaviors, or behaviors like flapping one's arms repeatedly, are typical behaviors for autistic people.

When it comes to communication, each person with ASD has a different set of skills. Some can speak well, while others may not be able to speak at all or only capable of speaking very little. Delayed speech and language skills, unrelated answers to questions, lack of pointing or response to pointing, and talking in flat tones are all signs that your child may have ASD. Autistic people that are capable of speech may use language in unconventional ways. They may not be able to use their vocabulary to form real sentences or say one word at a time. Others will repeat the same phrases or words repeatedly, and some children might repeat what they have heard others say, which is called echolalia. The repeated word may be spoken immediately or later.

For instance, you might say to your child, "Do you want some juice?" to which they may reply, "Do you want some juice?" rather than answering the question. While many non-ASD children also go through an echolalia stage, it generally passes by the time they are three years old. Some individuals with ASD might be able to speak clearly but may experience difficulty listening to what the people around them say. They might experience trouble understanding and using body language, gestures, or tone of voice. For instance, children with autism may not understand what waving goodbye means, and their facial expressions, gestures, and movements might not correspond to what they are saying. Your child may smile when saying something sad or upsetting.

WHAT *ISN'T* ASD?

As awareness and knowledge of autism grows, so do the myths. As you have already learned, autism is currently diagnosed according to the behaviors that fit into three general categories: communication impairments, social difficulties, and patterns of repetitive, restrictive behaviors and interests. The associated challenges can be obvious, such as stereotypical motor movements or language delays. Still, some deficits can be far more subtle and only show themselves in social situations, like problems with initiating conversations or play.

One of the most common myths about autism is that children with ASD will not look at you. Of course, we have already discussed that an irregular eye gaze is typical amongst many individuals with autism, but it is not a universal ASD experience. Neurotypical developing children will generally look into your eyes on instinct when talking to you, which can help them understand your feelings and gain meaning during social interactions. Some children with ASD might not look into a person's eyes intuitively when talking and instead focus on different parts of the body or face to receive meaning. Studies have suggested that people with autism do not have this social instinct due to their brain's underlying circuitry, which is generally different from neurotypicals.

Another common myth is that children with ASD have no interest in social interaction. This is untrue, and in fact, most children with autism are eager to make friendships, have friends, and interact socially, but generally experience difficulty knowing how to do so. Social graces are a luxury that naturally comes to neurotypical people and not to children with autism, meaning that you will often need to teach your child the hidden social rules. This can be done by role-playing activities with parents, peers, or carers or structured learning programs. Due to their inherent social awkwardness, children with ASD can become socially withdrawn and anxious, despite wanting social contact and friendship. This is generally a lifelong problem for those with autism.

Many people believe that children with autism are not affectionate, which again is untrue. ASD children are more than capable of expressing affection, and they do so frequently, though this expression may vary from neurotypical children due to unusual responses to sensory stimuli. ASD children could be oversensitive to hugs or touch, for instance, but may have a high threshold for pain. ASD children are often perceived as detached, but this does not indicate a lack of interest in affection but rather may be underpinned by a desire to engage in something that they find more interesting. Likewise, some children with ASD may not understand the purpose of hugging or why people shake hands and will need to be taught this social convention.

One of the most harmful myths about ASD is that boys and girls experience different core symptoms of autism. There is no consistent evidence - there's barely any evidence at all - that the core symptoms of autism are different in boys and girls, but there is a trend for girls to experience fewer stereotyped and restricted behavioral patterns than boys.

For instance, boys tend to line up their toys in order of color and size more than girls. Any differences may have a basis in biology, but they might also be due to the different ways that boys and girls are socialized. Gender stereotypes would have us believe that girls are better at socialization and communication, while boys are louder and more aggressive. These stereotypes may affect how the two sexes develop, and research in this area has yet to uncover the contribution of nurture versus nature, though any differences tend to be small. Most studies found that girls and boys experience similar ASD symptoms of similar severity.

The fifth and final myth I'll discuss is that autism is the same thing as Asperger's. These two disorders were previously defined as separate conditions that fit under the Pervasive Developmental Disorders umbrella term. Asperger's disorder was considered different from autism in that the development of language in the affected individual must have been within typical milestones, of single words by two years of age, phrase speech by three. Their intellectual capability would also have to have been within the normal range. Children that had Asperger's may have presented as verbally precocious 'little professors' and were often not assessed until they had entered a socially-charged environment like elementary school, where social differences become more apparent.

On the other hand, children with ASD were generally diagnosed earlier in life due to language delays and more characteristic autistic behaviors. However, as we have already discussed, the DSM-5 dissolved the distinction between autism and Asperger's, with both falling under the term Autism Spectrum Disorder. While this presented several challenges for diagnosis and treatment to ensure that ASD children receive the specialized care they need, it also made testing and diagnosis more accurate.

Chapter references

Hodges, H., Fealko, C., & Soares, N. (2020). Autism spectrum disorder: definition, epidemiology, causes, and clinical evaluation. *Translational Pediatrics*, 9(Suppl 1), S55–S65. https://doi.org/10. 21037/tp.2019.09.09

Autism Spectrum Disorder. (n.d.). MedlinePlus. Retrieved February 12, 2021, from https://medlineplus.gov/autismspectrumdisorder. html#:%7E:text=Autism%20spectrum%

20disorder%20(ASD)%20is,syndrome%20and%20pervasive%20developmental%20disorders

Basics About Autism Spectrum Disorder (ASD) | NCBDDD | CDC. (2020, March 25). Centers for Disease Control and Prevention. https://www.cdc.gov/ncbddd/autism/facts.html

Hodges, H. (2015, February 26). *Signs & Symptoms | Autism Spectrum Disorder (ASD) | NCBDDD | CDC.* Centers for Disease Control and Prevention. https://www.cdc.gov/ncbddd/autism/signs.html

May, T., & Rinehart, N. (2012, March 20). *Five myths about autism.* The Conversation. https://theconversation.com/five-myths-about-autism-4203

NIMH » Autism Spectrum Disorder. (2021, February 12). National Institute of Mental Health. https://www.nimh.nih.gov/health/topics/autism-spectrum-disorders-asd/index.shtml

2

UNIQUE CHALLENGES THAT ASD CHILDREN FACE

Many practitioners and laypeople focus on the autism of autism spectrum disorder, but the word 'spectrum' is arguably the most important word in the phrase. It was first used scientifically in the field of optics to describe the rainbow of colors in visible light and illustrates the vast level of diversity amongst patients with Autism Spectrum Disorder. 'Spectrum' reflects the wide array of skills, symptoms, and levels of impairment and challenges that children with ASD can present and face. Sometimes, symptoms may manifest as mild impairment for some individuals while causing severe disability for others.

Most children with ASD are highly intelligent. As a matter of fact, the intellectual ability of 46% of children with ASD is above average or average, according to the CDC (Centers for Disease Control and Prevention). 'Spectrum' also indicates that there are no two people with ASD in this world that are alike. While everyone with the disorder generally struggles with social skills, communication, and flexibility of thought, each child has a unique set of characteristics that make their ASD slightly different from another's. Even two siblings with ASD can be significantly different.

If you've met one person with autism, you've met one person with autism. In this chapter, we'll be taking a look at some of the unique challenges that children with ASD face, whether they're at home, in the classroom, or with their friends.

DIFFICULTY IN THE CLASSROOM

School is rarely a good environment for children with ASD, which is a problem for two reasons. The first is that children with ASD spend a lot of their time learning how to cope with an environment that is not suited to their challenges and abilities, and after having struggled to grow those skills over the years, they are forced to leave that environment to move to a totally different situation once they graduate or age out. For many children on the spectrum, school is way more challenging than any work environment for a number of spectacular reasons. Unfortunately, it seems that any ordinary public school in the 21st century has been designed to make life uncomfortable and highly difficult for children with even the mildest of challenges.

Sensory dysfunction - When it comes to sensory dysfunction, even children that have a mild over-reaction to bright lights, loud noise, and other sensory inputs are almost guaranteed to become nervous as a result of fluorescent lights, loud buzzers, echoing gyms, noisy children, and many other sights and sounds that are commonplace at public school.

Reading or speech comprehension - Difficulty with reading and speech comprehension is another challenge that children with autism will struggle to overcome at public school. Standardized testing and 'rigor' mean that even very young children are expected to be able to comprehend and respond to written and spoken language at top speeds. As children age, generally older than 7, any hint of visual or hands-on learning evaporates, and verbal expectations are placed even higher. Children with ASD are pretty much certain to be at a major disadvantage, as verbal understanding and expression are areas of difficulty for them.

Executive functioning - Children with autism generally also experience difficulty with executive functioning at school. Executive functioning is the ability to plan and execute multi-step projects, keeping in mind things like timeline, project parameters, and various other factors. In other words, it entails the ability to manage school projects, homework, studying for tests, and planning ahead for field trips, summer opportunities, and other events. Executive functioning is something that is expected of students throughout the school year, which of course, puts children on the spectrum at yet another disadvantage.

Social communication difficulties - Of course, you already know that autistic individuals at all stages of life experience difficulty with social communication. Sometimes these challenges can be very severe and obvious, but even for children with ASD that display good language skills, thinking socially can be quite difficult. At school, there will always be social challenges lurking around the corner, and they are always in flux. What might be appropriate in the halls is wholly inappropriate in the classroom. At the same time, what is appropriate on the playground would be totally unacceptable in the gym. It can be extremely difficult for children with autism to tell bullying from playful teasing or recognize humor or sarcasm. Even if a child with ASD is able to master appropriate social skills in the 1st grade, the rules will change in the summer and once again in the fall, leading to major confusion.

Fine and gross motor challenges - Fine motor skills are incredibly important for drawing, writing, pasting, cutting, and manipulating small objects like tweezers and glass slides. On the other hand, gross motor skills are used when running, jumping, throwing, kicking, and skipping. Moderate to mild problems in these areas, which most individuals with ASD face, can create major challenges on the playground, in the classroom, and on the playing field, amongst many other school-related environments. Motor planning, such as, "How hard should I throw? Can I jump down there safely?", is another related, important challenge.

Difficulty with changes in schedules and routines - Children with autism thrive on routines, but even throughout the school year, ensuring consistency in schedules and routines can be problematic in the school setting. From teacher training days to extended vacations, to snow days and assemblies, special events, standardized testing, and more, school schedules are targets that move non-stop. ASD children have the added burden of needing to leave classes, often in the middle of one, to attend social skills groups, therapy sessions, and other programs intended to help them handle the very experiences that they're skipping.

Lack of tolerance for autistic passions and behaviors - You would think that, in the world we live in today, teachers would understand and accept the fact that children learn and behave in different ways. However, in many cases, you'd be wrong. Sometimes it is because a particular teacher finds it distracting or upsetting to have a student who flicks, rocks, or moves in otherwise unexpected ways, talks too much about a certain interest, or experiences difficulty collaborating with their peers. Often a teacher is handicapped by their expectation that their class will make progress at a predetermined rate and respond to standardized test questions in a predetermined format within a predetermined time.

Difficulties with changing expectations and rules - As learners return to school every fall, they find that some things have not changed, while others have. Teacher A has no problem with students getting up to stretch, while Teacher B will not tolerate any of this behavior. Teacher A wants all students to show their work, while Teacher B only wants to see that their learners are getting the correct answers. Changes in peer behaviors can be even more challenging than changes in teacher expectations. Things like changes in interactions, norms, expectations, cultural preferences, clothing styles, and even word choices amongst peers can be nightmarish for ASD children.

The bottom line is that most modern schools were not designed with universal access in mind, but were rather designed for a particular demographic of students - those who do not face any of the challenges mentioned above. For students with any sort of differences, there are 'special' accommodations, which often consist of 'separate but equal' activities, classrooms, and even curricula. For ASD students, school can be the most challenging setting of them all. This is a problem in and of itself, as for most autistic students, the outside of a classroom is the only place that their real interests, abilities, and talents can be seen.

These are but a few of the numerous challenges that children with ASD face in the classroom and at school, which is why finding an autism advocate, or being your child's own advocate, is so important. They need the representation at school to ensure that all of their needs are being met and that they are receiving a quality education that caters to their unique challenges.

DIFFICULTY RELATING TO NON-ASD PEERS

Understanding the nature of the relationships that children with ASD have with their peers requires a multi-faceted approach. A good starting point is to consider social actions - a shared process in which children react to and initiate social stimulation from their peers, which fosters the development of peer relationships. Naturalistic studies conducted on social interaction patterns in autism both during childhood and adolescence have resulted in several common findings.

For starters, children with ASD often experience lower quality and quantity of social interactions than their neurotypical peers. They are generally far less likely to accept or initiate social interactions with their peers and spend more time engaging in solitary behaviors. These differences are true even when compared to children that have non-ASD disabilities. ASD peer interaction appears to be unrelated to the level of functioning, though early nonverbal communication and play skills might predict the extent of engagement with peers. Some evidence has suggested that the frequency of interaction is not affected when adults, rather than peers, are the target.

There is very little research regarding peer awareness, understanding of, and attitudes toward children on the spectrum from their neurotypical peers. But there is some evidence out there that provides some insight into the way children with autism are treated by their peers. First and foremost, younger children have proven to be the most accepting of disability, but otherwise, there is no obvious age-related trend. Secondly, it is important to note that social contact moderates attitudes. For instance, children that attend inclusive schools display more positive attitudes toward disabilities than children that do not attend inclusive schools.

Girls appear to be more accepting of disability than boys, though this is moderated by the sex of the attitudinal target. Finally, when it comes to awareness, children generally show a deeper understanding of physical and sensory disabilities than those that are considered to be 'hidden', or that display no obvious physical signs. Thanks to this significant evidence suggesting that children with ASD and young people experience reduced frequency and quality of interaction with their peers, we can safely say that this is driven both by lack of understanding and awareness and established social difficulties amongst peers.

Because of this, children with autism are often segregated from important sources of social support in the microsystem of the peer group, which makes them more vulnerable to victimization and bullying. In a 2010 study, it was found that adolescents with ASD that attended mainstream schools reported significantly lower social support from both friends and classmates than children with other or no disabilities. The study also significantly demonstrated that social support from classmates acted as a protective buffer against victimization and bullying. The peer relationships that children on the spectrum have have been scrutinized closely by researchers in the past twenty years and most studies have pointed out the differences from learners with no or other disabilities that converge into a general profile of negative experiences with peers. Conversely, a small but expanding field of research has begun to consider peer understanding, awareness, and attitudes toward Autism Spectrum Disorder.

This research has proven that understanding and awareness of autism has increased in recent years but still remains at a relatively low level. Attitudes tend to vary as a function of the extent to which information explaining the nature of autism is provided to non-ASD children and adolescents and how said information is presented and communicated.

Children with ASD are more likely to be the target of bullying amongst their peers than children who do not have autism. This is due to the fact that children that bully generally target children that are shy, quiet, and lack friendship skills - traits that nearly all children with autism will display or appear to display. Bullies also tend to target children who behave differently or express different interests, styles, and trends from themselves and other children in the same age group. Additionally, children with autism may not know how to join a group and might act in ways that neurotypical people would consider inappropriate, such as displaying attention-seeking behavior, wrestling, or dominating. Other children may be annoyed or upset by this, which can lead to verbal or physical clashes with peers. These are hardly ever resolved quickly. How do you explain to a 3rd grader that the ASD child didn't mean it?

Children with ASD may also experience determining which peers would be beneficial to spend time with and which peers would be detrimental. In other words, they may be less likely to avoid children that bully on the playground and unintentionally subject themselves to bullying. They may also believe most of what they are told - "If you do this, I'll be your friend".

Bullying is something that most children with ASD are susceptible to, especially during the later stages of elementary school and throughout high school. In the next section, we'll discuss the dangers of bullying and alienation that ASD children face when at school and what you can do to support your child.

ALIENATION & BULLYING

What is it that makes children on the spectrum vulnerable to bullying? An inability to communicate particular feelings and thoughts is the primary factor. While bullying is not an uncommon occurrence at school, even for children that have not been diagnosed with ASD, there are certain characteristics that ASD children display that make them easier targets for bullying. Children with autism may show limited control over their situations and the things that happen around them, experience poor self-esteem and feelings of inadequacy, be socially alienated from their peers, and appear self-destructive or depressed.

Because many children with ASD find it difficult to understand the tone of voice or body language of their peers, they may not even realize when they are being bullied. What's more, because they are unable to communicate certain thoughts and feelings accurately, they may unknowingly offend a classmate or peer and set themselves up for bullying. Children with autism are generally unable to defend themselves verbally, cannot solve problems, and may not be able to relate episodes of bullying in words. Bystanders such as teachers, peers, and parents are the ones with all the power to stop the bullying. More than 50% of bullying instances cease due to intervention.

Outbursts that children on the spectrum may display can be seen as disruptive or frightening by peers, despite being a result of unbearable levels of anxiety and stress. It is also a challenge for other children to understand some of the common differences that children with ASD have, such as having a particular sensitivity to noise or a high passion for certain interests. Jokes and sarcasm, as we have discussed, can be problematic for children with ASD, as they tend to take the literal meaning of what is said. For instance, a teacher may say to a child with autism, "You need to pull up your socks.", when intending to encourage more effort. The child may become confused and respond with what is perceived to be a cheeky or inappropriate response when all they did was act on the literal meaning of the comment.

As adolescence approaches, social conventions and groupings become more complex and important, presenting even more challenges. While bullying is generally believed to decrease with age, research has suggested that this may not be the case for young people with autism. We should be more concerned, rather than less, as this group of young people ages. There have been several tragic cases where a young person with autism has taken their own life, often as a result of years of isolation and bullying from their peers. While this is thankfully a rare occurrence, the short and long-term effects of falling victim to bullying have been well-documented. These consequences include difficulties at school, low self-esteem and self-worth, and mental health issues, all of which can persist long after the bullying has stopped.

All of these things paint quite a somber picture, but it is essential to remember that not all young ASD individuals are bullied, and there are strategies that can be implemented to prevent and avoid it. So, how can you help your child avoid bullying? The answer is not difficult. As a parent, there are a few ways you can help your ASD child, or any other ASD child for that matter, from being bullied. You can start by letting school officials know if you hear about your child or another child being bullied. They will be able to mediate the situation and react accordingly by supporting your child and the bully with the appropriate punishment.

Bullying is a complex, context-based problem, and it's important that you don't take on one aspect in isolation but rather develop adaptive strategies. Nevertheless, we must not only focus on the victims but the bullies and bystanders as well. There is evidence that teaching students what to do when they encounter bullying can help protect victims, as children can learn how to intervene, pressure the bullies, and seek the assistance of an adult. Teachers that have a keen awareness of autism can be vital in encouraging difference and individuality and promoting tolerance. It is also essential to achieve a balance between independence and support at school.

Too much support from adults - yes, it's a thing - can prevent children with autism from experiencing appropriate and important contact with their peers. On the other hand, a lack of support can lead to increased vulnerability to bullying, such as at break/lunchtime or on the school bus. Close collaboration and contact between school and home and also help foster positive relationships, and it is valued by parents, who might be the first to identify the warning signs that their child has fallen victim to bullying.

OTHER DISORDERS THAT SOMETIMES ACCOMPANY ASD

Children diagnosed with Autism Spectrum Disorder can also be born with a number of other conditions, which are called co-occurring conditions. These can appear at any stage during childhood, and some may not appear until adolescence or adulthood. The accompanying conditions can often make the life of an ASD child more challenging, and while they are generally few and far between, it is essential to know what conditions your ASD child may also have and how they can affect their day-to-day lives.

One of the most common conditions that children with autism have is anxiety. Individuals with anxiety experience a range of symptoms, including restlessness, tension, worry, hyperactivity, and fear. For children with autism, anxiety can manifest as stimming - unusual, repetitive movements - more often, asking questions repeatedly, having trouble falling asleep, or hurting themselves. About 40%-60% of children with ASD suffer from anxiety, with social anxiety being one of the most common anxiety disorders. Social anxiety generally occurs because children on the spectrum have difficulties in social situations that can make them feel stressed. Behavior therapy, relaxation techniques, and cognitive behavior therapy can all be used to treat anxiety in children with autism, though some children may also require medication.

Another condition that children on the spectrum experience is Attention Deficit Hyperactivity Disorder or ADHD. While many children often fail to think before they act and struggle to sit still and focus, children with ADHD experience the extreme versions of these behaviors, which have a major effect on their daily lives. The behaviors generally occur simultaneously, though some children can mainly be inattentive. Autism and ADHD share some common characteristics, such as not seeming to listen when others are speaking, intruding on the personal space of others, and interrupting. Many children with ASD display behavior that is very similar to the behavior of children with ADHD. While there is no cure, children and teenagers can learn to manage their symptoms through medication, behavior strategies, or a combination of both.

Bipolar disorder is a psychiatric condition that some ASD individuals may suffer from. People with bipolar disorder experience both extreme emotional highs, or mania, and extreme emotional lows, or depression. Depression is generally quite obvious, with the affected individual displaying a lack of motivation, low mood, poor appetite, and trouble sleeping, while mania is generally more difficult to spot. Its symptoms include reduced need for sleep, extreme self-esteem, more talking, and higher levels of activity than usual. Children with autism, and neurotypical children as well, that have bipolar disorder will exhibit big and fast changes in behavior and mood. When they go through these changes in mood, they may also have difficulty paying attention, behaving appropriately, and sitting still. There has not been much research into autism and bipolar disorder, but studies have suggested that it is not very common in young children on the spectrum. Treatment is generally long-term, often involving medication and behavior treatments.

Clinical depression is another condition that your child with ASD may suffer from. Its symptoms include poor sleep and appetite, low mood, a loss of motivation, and irritability. In children, symptoms of depression can also be cranky moods rather than just low moods and sadness. Depression can be quite common amongst children with autism, especially amongst those that are aware of their social difficulties. ASD individuals may be more likely to have symptoms of depression if they also have more severe symptoms of autism, are older, and display a greater verbal IQ. Medical professionals use a combination of psychotherapy, such as cognitive-behavioral therapy, and medication to treat depression. The effectiveness of the treatment is dependent on several factors, including the individual's optimism, experience with other treatments, and control over things that bring them stress. It also depends on how long the individual has been suffering from depression and how much their family and friends support them. One important thing to note is that CBT is a talking therapy, meaning that it will not be effective with children and adolescents that do not or cannot use language to communicate.

Down syndrome can also accompany autism and is a genetic disorder. While the majority of people are born with 23 pairs of chromosomes, people with Down syndrome - also called Trisomy 21 - are born with an additional 21st chromosome. This causes characteristic developmental delays, facial features, poor muscle tone, intellectual disadvantages, potential vision and hearing problems, and congenital heart defects. Down syndrome can be identified with tests during pregnancy, and if it is not detected then, it will generally be diagnosed at birth or in the child's early infancy. Only a small number of children are also born with Down syndrome. This is because the syndrome is quite uncommon, occurring only in 1 in every 1 100 births. On the other hand, autism is relatively common in children that have Down syndrome, and up to 40% of children that are born with Down syndrome are also born autistic. Down syndrome can be treated quite effectively to ensure that the affected individual experiences the best quality of life possible.

Finally, intellectual disability and developmental delays can sometimes accompany autism. It can be diagnosed when a child that is at least 6 years old has an IQ below 70, as well as difficulties with day-to-day tasks. In children under 6 years, the term 'developmental delay' is used when they experience significant delays in language and cognizance.

Intellectual disability will vary from person to person, and children on the spectrum with intellectual disabilities may have an uneven set of skills, meaning that they may be some things they are very good at, while other things they find difficult. For most cases, ASD children will experience the most difficulty with verbal skills, such as speech, listening, and comprehension - more so than with nonverbal skills like drawing or doing puzzles.

Chapter references

Conditions that can occur with autism. (2021, February 12). Raising Children Network. https://raisingchildren.net.au/autism/learning-about-autism/about-autism/conditions-that-occur-with-asd

Friends and peers: children and teenagers with autism spectrum disorder. (n.d.). Raising Children Network. Retrieved February 15, 2021, from https://raisingchildren.net.au/autism/communicating-relationships/connecting/friends-peers-asd#:%7E:text=Children%20with%20autism%20spectrum%20disorder%20(ASD)%20are%20-more%20likely%20to,shy%20and%20lack%20friendship%20skills.

Furfaro, H. (2020, May 7). *Autism health — Conditions that accompany autism, explained.* Spectrum | Autism Research News. https://www.spectrumnews.org/news/conditions-accompany-autism-explained/

Hebron, J. (2014, June 30). *Why children with autism often fall victim to bullies.* The Conversation. https://theconversation.com/why-children-with-autism-often-fall-victim-to-bullies-27087

Hetzler, L. (2020, September 1). *The Challenges of the Autism Spectrum*. Relias. https://www.relias.com/blog/the-challenges-of-the-autism-spectrum

Jo Rudy, L. (2020, August 3). *Good Reasons Why Your Autistic Child Has a Tough Time With School*. Verywell Health. https://www.verywellhealth.com/why-school-is-so-challenging-4000048

Morewood, G. D. (2020, April 5). *Autism and peer relationships | Optimus Education Blog*. The Optimus Blog. https://blog.optimus-education.com/autism-and-peer-relationships#:%7E:text=With%20significant%20evidence%20indicating%20that,and%20understand-ing%20(and%20subsequent%20exclusionary

Stimming: autistic children and teenagers. (2020, November 19). Raising Children Network. https://raisingchildren.net.au/autism/behaviour/common-concerns/stimming-asd

3

THE SECRETS TO COMMUNICATING WITH YOUR CHILD WITH ASD

Now for the part you picked up this book for - the secrets to communicating with your ASD child. As we have discussed throughout the previous chapters, communication is something that children with autism struggle with, as they find it difficult to understand others' tone of voice, facial expressions, and intentions. They can find it challenging to relate to other people and are generally slower to develop language skills, have significant difficulty understanding and using spoken language, or have no language at all. Your child may not understand that communication is a two-way street that makes use of facial expressions, eye contact, gestures, and of course, words - it's a good idea to keep these things in mind when teaching them language skills.

Children with ASD often appear self-absorbed, and as though they are living in their own private world in which they have limited ability to communicate and interact with others successfully. The ability that they have to communicate and make use of language is dependent on their social and intellectual development - some ASD children may be unable to communicate using language or speech, while some may develop very limited speaking skills. Others may develop rich vocabularies and be capable of talking about and describing certain objects in great detail, though many children with autism will have trouble with the rhythm and meaning of words and sentences. They may also be incapable of understanding the meaning of different vocal tones and body languages. All in all, the challenges hinder the ability of children with ASD to interact with others, especially individuals their age.

Some children with ASD may develop good, comprehensible speech but may still struggle to learn how to use language to communicate with others. They may also communicate mostly to protest something or ask for something, rather than for social reasons, such as for getting to know someone or making friends. How well children with ASD are able to communicate is important for other areas of their development, like learning and behavior. Without a good basis of communication, it will be difficult to teach your child to overcome some of the other challenges that they may face in their life.

In this chapter, you'll learn the secrets to being able to communicate with your ASD child.

HOW ASD SPEECH & LANGUAGE PROBLEMS ARE TREATED

As we mentioned previously, if a doctor suspects that a child has Autism Spectrum Disorder or any other developmental disability, they will generally refer the child to a number of specialists, including a speech-language pathologist. Speech-language pathologists are professionals that are trained to treat individuals with speech, voice, and language disorders. They will perform a comprehensive assessment of the child's ability to communicate, which will then create an appropriate treatment program. Additionally, the speech-language pathologist may make a referral for a hearing test to ensure that the child can hear normally.

As you know, in order for a child with ASD to achieve their full potential when they grow up, it is important that they are taught to improve their communication skills. There are a number of different approaches to this, but the best treatment programs start early, during preschool years, and are tailored to the unique needs of the child. The program should address both the child's communication skills and behavior and offer regular actions of positive reinforcement. Nearly all children with ASD respond well to specialized, highly-structured programs, and parents or caregivers, as well as other family members, should be involved in the treatment program so that it becomes a regular part of the child's everyday life.

For some younger children with autism, improving language and speech skills is a realistic treatment goal. Parents can increase their child's chance of achieving this goal by monitoring their development of language early on - just as toddlers learn to crawl before they can walk, children, ASD children included, must first develop their pre-language skills before they are able to start using words. These skills include things like using gestures, eye contact, imitation, body movements, babbling, and other vocalizations to aid in communication. Children that do not have these skills may be assessed and treated by a speech-language pathologist for further delays in development.

For slightly older ASD children, communication training teaches the basic language and speech skills, like single words and short phrases. Advanced training places emphasis on the way that language serves a purpose, like learning to hold a conversation with someone, which involves staying on a certain topic and taking turns when speaking. Some children on the spectrum may never develop their oral language and speech skills, and for these children, the goal would be to learn how to communicate using gestures, like sign language. For others, the goal might be to communicate using a symbol system with pictures used to express thoughts and feelings. Symbol systems can range from picture cards and boards to advanced electronic devices that generate speech through the use of buttons to represent common actions or items.

TEACHING YOUR CHILD TO MANAGE & COPE WITH THEIR ANGER

Some of the underlying characteristics of ASD can lead to behavioral problems like frustration and angry outbursts in children. One such characteristic is the inability to communicate and express one's thoughts and feelings to others, which often leads to frustration and feelings of being ignored or misunderstood. Another may be the tendency for a child with autism to require 'sameness', with no changes to alterations to their routine - any changes in the familiar surroundings or daily schedule can provoke anxiety and lead to upset. Calming a child with ASD down can be exhausting and stressful, but it is important to know how to deal with these outbursts and manage them constructively.

If you want to deal with your child's anger effectively, you will first need to determine where it's coming from. This can be quite a challenge, especially if they struggle to communicate their feelings and desires to you. Ask your child what's wrong, and pay close attention to what they are telling you or trying to get you to understand. Help them learn to process and manage their anger through communication. Are they upset because they can't find their favorite object or toy? Or is it something deeper? Try your best to understand what is causing your child to be frustrated. You might notice that temper tantrums occur at the same time every day, which could be a clue to the trigger.

One of the useful and important tools that you can use in situations where your child is angry or frustrated, but experiencing difficulty with expressing their emotions, is a communication strategy or device. You can develop a kind of visual representation or board of triggers, emotions, and consequences to help your child express themselves. Once you have identified the trigger, you have the opportunity to avoid it in the future. Give your child some time to express their feelings, and make sure that they know that you care about what they are feeling. Stay calm, and above all else, resist the urge to raise your voice at them - modeling good behavior for your child to learn from is one of the most valuable things you can do. Perhaps the problem is something that can be remedied with ease, but then again, the source of frustration may be something that you do not have control of. In this case, changing the immediate surroundings, or trying to shift your child's focus onto something else, can help you ease their anger.

When rage becomes unavoidable, it is essential that your child has a safe place to vent their feelings, where they will not be able to harm themselves or anyone else. You can try directing their anger by offering them a soft object, like a pillow, to scream in or use as a punching bag. After a while, they will have let out their frustration and tired themself out, and will be calmer. Another way to allow your child to express themself is to encourage them to write down their feelings in a journal if they are able, or talk about the thing that is bothering them. A great way to allow them to express their emotions is through art, so encourage them to draw a picture or write a poem. By teaching your child that there are safe ways for them to express all of their emotions, even the negative ones, you will help them learn to manage their anger in a more constructive way.

You should also set a safe space in your home where your child can calm themself down. This could be their playroom or bedroom, and you should ensure that the designated area is safe and does not house things that could break or otherwise harm someone if knocked over or thrown. You can set this safe spaces' mood and fill it with all of the things that your child finds soothing and pleasant. Try to create an ambiance that is more subdued by making the area quieter or less bright, which is especially useful if your child suffers from sensory overload. It is important to remember that not all children with autism have the same preferences or triggers, so experiment to find out what works best for calming your child down. One child might find the sunlight soothing, while another may dislike it and prefer the curtains drawn.

When your child can't get what they want, you should attempt to reach a compromise. If they are angry because they can't have or do something that they want at that moment, try to reach a compromise, if appropriate. Perhaps they want to have dessert before eating dinner - tell them that if they finish their dinner, you'll make them an extra special dessert or give them a bigger serving than usual. They might also enjoy baking and decorating cookies with you or making an ice cream sundae. You should not just give in to your child's demands to stop their bad behavior - for children below the age of 8 years old, a period of time out for bad behavior can be effective, and teach them that they cannot be rewarded for misbehaving. You should also always praise and reward your child for their good behavior and for following the rules; a little bit of positive reinforcement can go a long way in managing their anger. It can be something as simple as rewarding them with a star sticker on a chart for their good behavior, where they receive a special reward for collecting a certain number of stars.

If your child's anger leads to physical violence, you will need to talk to them about the possible consequences of such behavior and should never ignore violence. Even a small child can do some serious damage to others in a fit of rage, but they will someday be much bigger and become a significant safety issue. Let your child know that violent behavior will not be tolerated. There are serious consequences for violent people, such as juvenile detention or jail. Of course, we're not suggesting that you use scare tactics on your child - you should simply be honest with them about your expectations, and if you need help, you should seek professional help.

ADAPTING LOVE LANGUAGES

Just like any other parent, as a parent of a child or children with ASD, you want to express your unconditional love and support for your child. In fact, the feeling of being unable to express care and love is one of the largest frustrations that parents of children on the spectrum experience. How are you meant to express affection to your child who doesn't like to be touched? How do you give your child praise and affirmation when they aren't verbal. Or how are you supposed to show any love at all when your child leaves the room when anyone enters?

These are all problems that many parents of ASD children face, but fortunately, there are ways to adapt the way you express your love in order to meet your child's needs. Let's take a look at the five Love Languages, as well as some suggestions for adjustments you can make when using them to interact with your child. First, we'll take a look at why it is important to express unconditional love to your child.

Every child is fueled by love, and every day, their love tank needs to be refilled. A full tank of love will provide your child with the emotional strength they need in order to make it through the day. Your unconditional love is the premium fuel that fills your child's love tank the quickest, takes care of them the best, and lasts the longest. This is especially true for children with ASD and other special needs, who might need more support and more expressions of love than neurotypical children.

Unconditional love is the "no matter what" kind of love. It carries the most powerful messages and helps your child feel calm, accepted, and supported. If you're like many other parents, then you're probably worried about coddling or spoiling your child, and while a failure to discipline or always caving to your child's demands can lead them to be misbehaved and spoiled, this has nothing to do with love. It is simply impossible to love your child too much or spoil them with love and go on and love your child.

As you know, children with ASD can have emotional, physical, behavioral, psychological, and developmental challenges, and I can't say for certain that love will solve all of these problems. But I can safely say that love is the foundation and that it will be much more challenging to address behaviors and other problems that children with ASD face and present if you have not first expressed unconditional acceptance and love.

Figuring out your ASD child's main love language is as simple as paying attention to their behaviors and asking a few key questions. You should try to gauge their level of engagement or reaction to each of the properties of the different love languages we will discuss shortly. For instance, if your child tends to produce a greater level of positive response when you pay them a compliment than when you try to assist them in one of their tasks, then their main love language could be 'words of affirmation'. Conversely, if your child tends to become triggered when met with physical touch from others, then chances are their main love language is not 'physical touch'. Let's now take a look at the five love languages and how you can implement them to show your child affection.

Words of Affirmation

What reaction does your child have to verbal praise, checklists/reinforcement systems, and verbal praise? To start experimenting with words of affirmation, repeat the things they are verbalizing or what you feel they are attempting to communicate, even when you feel unsure about what they are saying. For instance, if your child is nonspeaking, and they are pointing to a picture repeatedly, try telling them, "That's a really cool picture, you're right!", then take note of their reaction. Repetition indicates that you are paying attention, which will build a trust in them that it is safe to communicate with you. You should also constantly speak to your child through choices. Children that value words of affirmation will, of course, value words, so even if you aren't always receiving a reaction when talking about routines or offering choices in snacks, don't become discouraged. It all accumulates over time. Finally, you should offer spoken praise right after your child displays desirable behaviors - praise that emphasizes the desired behavior. In other words, use phrases like, "I love the way you cleaned the table and put your dishes in the sink on your own. You're awesome!".

Receiving Gifts

How does your child behave when working for rewards or reinforces, around birthdays and holidays, or when they give something to you or someone else? You should allow your child to choose what they earn as a reward for good behavior, whether it's after they have finished their chores at home or completed work at school so that they can feel valued and empowered. Just remember to set your expectations - for instance, "Finish this math problem, then you can go play video games." - so that your child knows what they must do in order to receive their preferred reward. You should also be making a big deal about them earning their rewards, as sometimes the recognition is better than the material gift itself. If it's the month of your child's birthday, then you could put a countdown on the calendar for the household to see. When it's the big day, ask if they'd like to put on a special outfit or if they would like you to tell people. Make them feel as though it is a day that heralds true celebration because it is.

Acts of Service

Take note of how your child responds to situations requiring them to ask for help or assistance with tasks like chores and homework. If they experience trouble when requesting help, assure them that you are there to provide them with all the help they need. It sounds silly, but even as grown adults, we have a hard time accepting the fact that we sometimes can't do some things on our own and need help from someone else, so a reminder can soothe ASD children that tend to be anxious. This can be done when they are busy with homework, tying their shoes, or heating up leftovers in the microwave. You should also assist with difficult or non-preferred tasks without actually doing the task for your child. It might be extremely difficult not to interfere when your child is faced with a challenging task, but it helps to remember that you are benefiting them so much more when you provide assistance rather than completely taking over. For instance, if their chore is to wipe the counters and tables, get a cloth and tell them that you will wipe the chairs since they are making the tables look so shiny. It can sometimes be the small displays of support that they need to help them push through the task.

Sometimes, flipping the script and asking your child for help can make them feel valued and needed. If you don't have a free hand, ask them to open the door for you, and make sure your "thank you" is a gracious one. If they're savvy with technology, ask them for some help with your phone. Children with autism deserve and need to see that we are also vulnerable and how their own acts of service benefit us in our day-to-day lives.

Quality Time

Finally, take note of how your child reacts when they have free time and can choose to do what they want, they have your undivided attention and are engaging in groups of various sizes. Try to dedicate ten minutes of quality time each day, engaging in an activity that they love, for one week, whether you're playing video games, doing puzzles, or drawing. Your undivided attention will mean the world to your child - you'll be able to learn about them, they will be able to learn about you, and you will become an encyclopedia of fun stories and random knowledge. If your child has a tendency to disengage in larger groups, ensure that they feel included by encouraging them to join in on a conversation or asking them if they'd like to join in an activity. When you can, you should try to insert them into peer conversations to help them improve their social skills that would otherwise be difficult for them to do so on their own.

Physical Touch

Gauge how your child responds to affection like hugs and kisses, as well as proximity to others when sitting or standing. You should be giving them sensory breaks, as children with ASD whose primary touch is love language might also suffer from sensory processing disorder. While the disorder varies from individual to individual, sensory breaks allow for proper access to touch in order to regulate your child's senses. Sensory breaks may be things like brushes, shoulder squeezes, and more. You should also be allowing your child to decide who they are with, whether they're picking who they're sitting with on the couch or which team they'd like to be on. Giving them the freedom of choice makes them feel heard and happy, though you should ensure that you review appropriate touch expectations beforehand.

CLEAR COMMUNICATION IS KEY

This may seem like a given, but it is worth mentioning anyway. As we have already discussed countless times, children on the spectrum struggle to communicate for any number of reasons. It's important that you can break through these barriers and achieve meaningful communication with your child.

To start, you will want to get visual. For nonspeaking children, images can benefit efforts to communicate – your child can use cards with pictures on them to request the things they need or want. Additionally, cards that help express feelings can help your child understand and express their emotions better. Visuals encourage children to interact with others, and this interaction can even evolve into language. The best part is that, as technology becomes more sophisticated, apps for tablets and smartphones can fulfill the same purpose as a physical image card, making things easier for both you and your child, thanks to various accessibility settings available on the modern devices of today.

Next, you should always say what you mean. Most children with ASD take the literal meaning when it comes to wording. Using things like idioms, sarcasm, or other figures of speech will only cause confusion. Speak plainly, and do not embellish your language. Conversely, children with autism might use vocabulary that they do not understand fully because they memorized the word from a book, adult speech, a movie, or a TV show. Remember that when your child repeats these words or phrases in an inappropriate context, you will have to try to find other clues to understand what they are trying to say. This is actually an encouraging sign, as it means that your child is imitating the language and developing their own skills – they just need some help connecting words to specific contexts.

You will need a lot of patience when teaching your child, but you should not rush to give your child what you know they need straight away. Children learn to develop their language skills by asking for an item they desire rather when receiving it automatically or when they gesture for it. In the same vein, talk to your child about their daily routine rather than rushing from task to task. Ensure that you're speaking slowly, allowing your child plenty of time to take in your words, formulate their response, and remember to use appropriate gestures when talking to them. Reward and praise your child for their attempts to learn from you.

This may seem odd, but in times of need, you have the option of turning to an animal. While a service animal certainly won't teach your child to speak, they can help children with ASD in various ways that can eventually lead to improved communication with others.

Firstly, they are able to reduce stress and calm children that may be overstimulated down. Overstimulation is one barrier to communication in terms of amplified, distracting sound, and an animal might be able to help your child focus on other people that may be trying to talk to them. Secondly, animals can offer ASD children a sense of acceptance – if your child is afraid to attempt speech because of possible failure, an animal can act as a reassuring presence. Finally, if your child struggles with empathy and socialization, animals can help them open their emotions up and increase their sensitivity to the way others feel.

GETTING PAST ATTENTION-SEEKING BEHAVIORS

One of the most challenging behaviors to discourage in a child with ASD is those used to seek attention. Many children on the spectrum engage in certain behaviors that are meant to garner reactions from parents, siblings, caregivers, or teachers, and these behaviors can be anything from silly to aggressive and oppositional in nature. In this section, we'll discuss how you can pinpoint these attention-seeking behaviors, figure out why your child is displaying them, and strategies for discouraging them.

It isn't always obvious that your child is engaging in attention-seeking behaviors, and there are a number of ways to determine if your child's behavior is meant to get your attention and reaction. If your child looks directly at you when performing bad behavior, engages in the behavior repeatedly when you do not react the first time, gets your attention before performing bad behavior, talks about the bad behavior while engaging in it, or reports undesirable behavior that you might not have seen, then your child may be trying to get your attention through their behavior.

The primary reason that your child performs attention-seeking behavior is, of course, to get your attention and the attention from adults. However, this behavior can also be the result of a number of other factors. Attention-seeking behaviors may help your child avoid doing things they do not want to do – for instance, if your child does not want to bathe, they may perform bad behavior because they know it will result in a 'talk' or some timeout, which will delay the bath. They may also perform attention-seeking behaviors out of sheer boredom. It is essential that you determine why your child is performing attention-seeking behavior before you try to discourage it.

There are a number of strategies you can use to decrease these behaviors effectively. The trick is to choose the ones that offer little to no attention to the actual behavior – you're not trying to ignore your child, but instead trying to ignore the behavior as much as possible, because when you respond to attention-seeking behavior, you are giving your child precisely what they want: attention.

To start discouraging attention-seeking behavior, you need to make sure that you aren't letting them get the better of you. These behaviors can be a nuisance, to say the least, and you might feel tempted to react or ask your child to cease the behavior repeatedly. Remind yourself that your attention is what your child is after, so it should be the last thing they receive. When you ignore attention-seeking behavior, leaving the room or turning your back can be useful, as long as your child will be safe when unsupervised. If you are removing privileges or toys to decrease the behavior, use the fewest number of words possible to tell your child what they lost. For instance, "You lost your dragon toy for hitting." Do not engage in any complaints or arguments about what was being removed. Stay as calm and collected as possible. We cannot stress this enough, as even sounding or looking upset might be what your child is looking for. Finally, ensure that you are praising your child as much as possible for their positive behaviors. Often, we focus on the undesirable behaviors too much and forget to praise them for their good behavior.

MORE STRATEGIES FOR CLEAR COMMUNICATION

Of course, every single child on the spectrum is special and unique, so a strategy that may work for one child may be ineffective for another. Useful strategies will depend on what your child finds motivating. In this section, we'll give you a number of general communication tips that you can try with your child to encourage the development of their language and communication skills. Once again, not all of these will work with every child, so find which one works best for you.

Maintaining Attention

Now, while we have just discussed how to discourage behaviors in your child that are meant to get your attention, it is still important that you are providing them with all of the attention they need, especially when they perform positive, desirable behaviors. Help your child pay attention to you when you are playing together – you can encourage them to make eye contact with you by holding their favorite object or toy near your eye and waiting for them to look at you before you hand it over. Try a fun game for the both of you, like rolling a ball or blowing bubbles, and wait a few seconds for eye contact before rolling the ball or blowing a bubble, and so on.

Social Interaction & Play

Most children, neurotypical and autistic alike, learn the basics of language through interaction and play with their caregivers in meaningful ways. Encourage your child to play with you, get on the ground face to face, and start talking. They will likely mimic your behavior, which will help build the foundation for effective and meaningful communication.

Follow Your Child's Lead

Talk with your child about what they are already playing with or paying attention to. When you do this, they will be more likely to listen to you and learn vocabulary because you are discussing something that they like. This can be a great way to teach them a word to add to their vocabulary, and you may even hear these words repeated to you later on!

Alternative & Argumentative Communication

Some ASD children are either behind in talking and require a system to aid them in learning a language while they are learning how to talk or might rely on an alternative form of communication that isn't speech. There are plenty of devices and tools out there to help, such as the Picture Exchange Communication System, or PECS, sign language, electronic devices like Tobii or GoTalk, or certain software. Your child's speech-language pathologist can recommend the system that will work best for your child, and you should be sure to use this system when attempting to communicate with them.

Add Structure

Research has proven that children with Autism Spectrum Disorder respond the best when they know what to expect, so having a structure or routine in place around the house can help them relax, which will allow them to learn more effectively. Putting a visual schedule up on the fridge depicting your routine at home can help your child learn to follow a schedule, avoid meltdowns, and learn the language and vocabulary associated not only with that routine but with other routines as well.

Social Thinking

For older children with ASD that are capable of speech and that have higher language levels, talking with others may be a challenge due to various social rules. They may have a difficult time knowing what these rules are, such as how to start a conversation, when one ends, how to keep the conversation going, or how to stay on topic. They may also experience difficulty understanding the other person's feelings or grasping their point of view. Explicitly explaining the 'rules of conversation' to your child and reading them books, and asking them to point out and interpret the feelings of the characters can be highly beneficial to them. Social language groups can also be a fantastic way to teach these skills and put them into practice.

Create a Team & Be a Member

Children with autism have special needs when it comes to language and speech, such as needing assistance with fine motor movements, managing unwanted behaviors, or managing sensory overload with lights and sounds, or seeking out sensory stimulation like turning on lights or making a noise. Getting help when addressing these problems from the right people can help your child learn language, as they will be in a better place to be motivated and pay attention. Behavioral consultants, occupational therapists, and other members of an allied health care team can provide help in these areas. You should also be a part of the team since practicing speech strategies at home and integrating them into your daily routine will make a world of difference. Parents are arguably the most important part of the team, and you are going to be the one to help your child reach their full potential.

Label Feelings as They Are Felt

What do I mean by this? Well, for instance, if your child is trying to get something to eat from the fridge, label the feeling by saying,

"You're hungry". The more your child is exposed to the word for that particular feeling and behavior, the better they will be able to understand the said feeling. This strategy must be a consistent one, and it needs to take place naturally. Modeling a feeling can happen when your child is happy, hurt, sad, excited, and so on. For example, as your child expresses their excitement, say to them, "I see you're quite excited!". If you have a picture of excitement, you can further reinforce the concept.

Enter Your Child's World Through Motivating Items & People

For a lot of children, food can be motivating. For others, it could be a certain friend, film, toy, neighbor, or family member. For instance, if your child loves spending time with a certain member of your family, you can 'use' this motivating person to encourage communication, and when you do so, you should use various auditory and visual strategies – use a picture of the family member and model their name. Encourage your child to point at the picture of the family member or exchange it with you to request it. When they are capable of pointing to or exchanging the picture, the motivating person can come over to your child and give them a hug to fulfill the request.

Assume That Your Child is Competent

This is one of the most important things you can do as a parent. Assuming that your child is competent is a form of empowerment, whether they have a disability or not. Assuming that your child can and will do what they need to is powerful and goes hand-in-hand with speaking to your ASD as you would with any other child.

Children with or without disabilities are very quickly able to detect when an adult or another child talks to them differently than they do to others. Talking to your child the way you would any other child, and encouraging others to do the same, will empower your child and inspire confidence in them, removing the feeling of 'otherness'.

Model Language

Modeling language is a fantastic strategy for promoting and encouraging communication and language-learning. Often, a child might not know a specific word or structure of a sentence. For example, if your child wants some juice at the dinner table, and is trying to indicate this desire to you, say "I want water," to them. Providing the model for them to learn from will improve your child's expressive and receptive language. Adding a word like "please" in a question form can also offer your child some clues as to the appropriate ways to ask for a certain item, which in turn will improve their pragmatic language skills.

Use a Total Communication Approach

When using a total communication approach, you should use aided and unaided communication. "What are those?" I hear you ask. Aided communication is communication via anything other than your body, including things like photographs. Many children with ASD are not capable of using speech for functional communication and will often use other systems of communication to express themselves. On the other hand, unaided communication is communication through body gestures, sign language, and facial expressions. The total communication approach is one of the best ways to communicate, as it includes all modes of communication – none of us talk just with speech. Sometimes, those around us can understand a complex message through a simple facial expression or gesture.

Chapter References

Ammacher, J. (2017, March 21). *Adapting the 5 Love Languages for children with autism.* Springbrook Autism Behavioral Health. https://springbrookautismbehavioral.com/portfolio-item/the-five-love-languages-and-children-with-autism/

Applied Behavior Analysis Programs Guide. (2017, October 17). *5 Ways to Communicate with Children with Autism.* https://www. appliedbehavioranalysisprograms.com/lists/5-ways-to-communicate-with-children-with-autism/

Autism Spectrum Disorder: Communication Problems in Children. (2020, December 14). NIDCD. https://www.nidcd.nih.gov/health/ autism-spectrum-disorder-communication-problems-children

Children's Support Solutions, Morneau Shepell. (2017, March 31). *Strategies to support speech development in children with ASD.* https://childrensupportsolutions.com/strategies-to-support-communication-development-in-children-with-asd/

Communication: children with autism spectrum disorder. (2020, May 14). Raising Children Network. https://raisingchildren.net.au/ autism/communicating-relationships/communicating/ communication-asd

Decreasing Attention-Seeking Behavior |. (2011, July 8). ACT. http://www.act4autism.com/decreasing-attention-seeking-behavior/

#:%7E:text=One%20of%20the%20most%20effective,be%20the%20very%20best%20strategy

Eisenberg, B. (2015, April 19). *5 Ways to Encourage communication with a Non Verbal Child Diagnosed with Autism - Friendship Circle - Special Needs Blog*. Friendship Circle -- Special Needs Blog. https://www.friendshipcircle.org/blog/2015/04/21/5-ways-to-encourage-communication-with-a-non-verbal-child-diagnosed-with-autism/

How To Manage Anger For Children With Autism. (2020, November 13). Lexington Services. https://lexingtonservices.com/how-to-manage-anger-for-children-with-autism/#:%7E:text=Let%20Your%20Child%20Express%20Anger%20In%20A%20Safe%20Place&text=Another%20way%20to%20let%20your,poem%20or%20drawing%20a%20picture

University of Rochester, Medical Center. (n.d.). *Interacting with a Child Who Has Autism Spectrum Disorder - Health Encyclopedia - University of Rochester Medical Center*. URMC. Retrieved February 19, 2021, from https://www.urmc.rochester.edu/encyclopedia/content.aspx?contenttypeid=160&contentid=46

Yassine, S. (2021, February 19). *How to Determine Your Child With Autism's Love Language*. The Mighty. https://themighty.com/2020/04/how-to-determine-child-with-autisms-love-language/

4

HOW TO HELP YOUR CHILD WITH AUTISM COMMUNICATE

Despite the fears that arise in parents of children with nonspeaking or minimal-language autism, researchers have published promising findings that, even after age 4, many nonspeaking children with ASD eventually develop language. While this language might not be the speech you're used to, with a little effort, you will still be able to understand it just the same and use it to communicate with your child. It's only natural for you as a parent to want to know how you can promote the development of language in your child with autism. Well, I have some good news: research has produced several effective strategies, and I'll be discussing these strategies throughout this chapter.

However, before we share these tips, it is vital that you remember that every child with autism is unique. Even with all the effort you can muster, a strategy that works perfectly for one child may not work for yours. Although every child with autism can learn to communicate, it isn't always through a spoken language. Nonspeaking individuals with autism are capable of much societal contribution and can lead fulfilling lives with the help of assistive technologies and visual supports.

In this chapter, we'll be taking a look at some of the best strategies for teaching your child with autism to communicate. Read on for more.

COMMUNICATION IN NONSPEAKING AUTISM

Children with nonspeaking autism experience the most difficulty when learning to communicate with others, as they do not have the luxury of using a spoken language to talk. Therefore, it's up to you as a parent to teach your child how to communicate through other means, whether it's through sign language, gestures, visual cues, or with the help of assistive technologies. Here are some strategies you can use to help your nonspeaking child with autism communicate.

Encourage Social Interaction & Play

Children learn a lot when they play, including language. Interactive play provides enjoyable, fun opportunities for you and your young one to communicate with each other by trying a wide range of games to find one that they enjoy. You should try playful activities that promote social interaction, such as reciting nursery rhymes, singing, and gentle roughhousing. During your interactions and play sessions with your child, position yourself in front of them and close to eye level so that it is easier for them to see and hear you.

Focus on Nonverbal Communication

This may seem like a given, but eye contact and gestures can build the foundation for language. Encourage your child by modeling and responding to these behaviors, exaggerating your gestures, and using both your voice and your body when communicating. For instance, extend your hand to point when you say, "Look", or nod your head when you say "Yes". Use gestures that your child will be able to imitate easily, including opening hands, clapping, outstretched arms, and so on. You should also be responding to the gestures that your child makes – when they look at a toy or point to it, hand it to her or take the cue and play with it. Similarly, point to a toy that you want, and either wait for your child to pick it up and hand it to you or pick it up yourself.

Imitate Your Child

Mimicking your child's play behaviors and sounds will encourage more interaction and vocalization. It will also encourage them to, in turn, copy you and take turns. Ensure that you are imitating how your child is playing, so long as it is positive behavior – for instance, when your child rolls a ball, you roll a ball as well. If they bounce their ball, you bounce yours too. Just remember only to imitate positive behavior!

Follow Your Child's Interests

Instead of interrupting your child's focus, follow along with them using words. Using the one-up rule, narrate what your child is doing. If they are playing with a shape sorter, you could say "in" when they put a shape in its correct slot. You could also say "shape" when they hold one of the shapes up and "dump shapes" when they dump the shapes out to start over. By talking about the things that engage your child and keeps them interested, you will help them learn the associated vocabulary.

Functional Communication Training

When children do not experience typically developing language skills, they may not have an effective way to express their needs and desires, resulting in the risk of them developing aggression, tantrums, or self-harming behaviors as a replacement. Not only are these behaviors potentially harmful, but they are often not understood.

This is where Functional Communication Training comes in. It involves teaching an individual with ASD a reliable way of conveying information in a number of ways, either through language, signs, or images – or a combination of all three – to achieve a desired end result. It is called 'functional' because its goal is not simply to teach children how to label an item (associating a picture of the word "yellow" to a banana) but rather aims to teach children to use words or signs to receive something they need or want, like a toy, food, an activity, a break from something, a trip to the bathroom.

Functional Communication Training involves using positive reinforcement to teach children about communication and language to improve their proficiency at effective interaction with others to meet their needs. So how does it work?

Stephanie Lee, one of the Child Mind Institute's clinical psychologists, has a great explanation for how a clinician implementing FCT works. According to Dr. Lee, they begin by identifying something that the child is highly motivated to achieve, like a favorite activity, toy, or food. This object will serve as the natural reward for using a picture or sign that represents that thing. So, if a child really loves Thomas the Tank Engine or Barbie, or their favorite food is cookies, the clinician would take that item and teach the child either a picture or sign that represents it.

The child is initially set up for something Dr. Lee calls 'errorless learning', in which the clinician guides them to use the picture or sign to obtain the reward. The form of supported communication is repeated, each time resulting in the reward being earned, until the child is capable of success with decreasing amounts of prompting from the clinician. As the prompting is reduced, the child becomes increasingly independent in their communication.

Once the child is able to use the word, sign, or picture for the item reliably when the item is present, the next step is generalization or using the word outside of the specific scenario that has been taught. For instance, if the child is watching TV and wants some cookies, they might use the sign they were taught to get the cookies, according to Dr. Lee. This kind of spontaneous use of the skill must also be reinforced over time, and after a particular sign or word is being used consistently, new ones may be added to build the child's repertoire. Once this system of communication has been learned – that the image or sign that they are using needs to be received by someone else in order for the child to receive the desired item – then a new picture or sign can steadily be introduced and taught.

So what are the goals with Functional Communication Training? Well, the rate at which a child progresses with the training will often depend on their cognitive level or level of functioning. For children that have a more significant language impairment or who have more complex needs, plenty of trials may be needed for them to grasp a handful of pictures or signs. They may end up with a small vocabulary of functional communication, but it is the vocabulary that they need the most, such as the foods they like, asking to use the bathroom, and so on.

Children that have less complicated needs and with a higher level of functioning may end up gaining just as much language, if not more, than their neurotypical peers. Some children will be able to speak complete sentences using an assistive technology device, which others will only gain single words. With the latter, a clinician would look to determine what goals would be the most appropriate. The benefit would be measured against the effort required to achieve said goal. Remember, treatment is catered to the specific abilities and needs of each child.

Functional Communication training is generally taught one-on-one with a clinician that is either a behavioral psychologist trained in Applied Behavior Analysis (ABA), or a speech-language pathologist. As a parent, you play an important role in reinforcing the training, practicing the things your child has learned and using it in a number of scenarios. When FCT takes place at school, teachers would be responsible for helping children practice the signs that they have learned.

Replacing Self-Injury With Language

Like all behavior, self-injury serves a function, usually to get attention, to escape an undesirable task, to get attention, or to serve a sensory need. When face slapping or head hitting results in a child receiving attention, receiving something they want, escaping an uncomfortable situation, or getting out of something they don't want to do, the behavior is being reinforced accidentally. Functional Communication Training can help break these unhealthy patterns in behavior. Once children have learned to ask for a break with either a word, picture or sign and get the results they desire efficiently and quickly, they are likely to choose the appropriate behavior rather than self-injury.

Functional Communication Training can and has been applied to individuals with ASD of all ages, from preschool to adulthood, but experts prefer to see it start as early as possible. Dr. Lee says that what we know about the development of language is that the earlier the intervention, the better, so the quicker we can build a child's communication repertoire, the better for them it will be. However, she also adds that she has seen FCT work exceptionally effectively with adults that did not experience training in their youth, and some gain skills rather quickly. She's also seen adults that took a very long time to develop a very small vocabulary, but even that small vocabulary was extremely important to them and to the people they were around when it comes to better understand the individual's wants and needs.

ASSISTIVE TECHNOLOGY

When children and older individuals with ASD have severe language and speech disabilities, alternative and augmentative communication strategies can provide them with an opportunity to express themselves and have a voice, as you have already learned throughout this chapter. We live in the age of ever-evolving technology, and one of tech's greatest advancements has to do with accessibility and assistance for those with disorders and disabilities. Those who were previously unable to hear can be fitted with hearing aids, and those who couldn't see can receive assistive sight technology. Those who couldn't talk can now speak through technology.

Being unable to communicate effectively has a significant impact on educational success, life, and the development of social skills and relationships. The frustrations that come with not being able to communicate can lead to negative behavior challenges as well, as you already know. Using devices like smartphones and tablets as an aid for communication in individuals with autism yields many benefits because they are portable and flexible, unlike other dedicated communication devices that can be cumbersome and heavy. Handheld devices are easily carried and can promote acceptance amongst peers, while the touchscreen and layout is more accessible for individuals with learning and coordination difficulties, as sliding and tapping are much easier than typing. Technology is able to improve communication with others simply by the timely use of texting or email, which has cost and time savings.

Research has found that, as new technology is developed and progress is made at an increasing rate each year, children's awareness and competency with technology also increases. Children's increasing use of technology implies both communicational and educational practices, as it is now a common part of their everyday environments and lives. Children are 'native' technology users, as it is something they have grown up with, which is often true for children with ASD. Many individuals on the spectrum are more comfortable when interacting with inanimate objects like tablets or computers, and many are also visual learners with strong technological skills. Until fairly recently, most tablets were used for gaming and entertainment purposes, and though the varied use of technology for ASD children continues to receive little to no attention, despite the fact that technology is generally a high-interest area for many of these children, we know that it can be used effectively not only for entertainment and as an assistive device, but also as a device to assist in teaching social skills, academics, reinforcement, video modeling, fine motor skills, speech and language therapy, functional life skills, visual supports, increasing independence, and organizational skills.

What Exactly is Assistive Technology, Exactly?

Assistive technology refers to any piece of equipment, item, or product system, whether acquired off the shelf, commercially, customized, or modified, that is used to maintain, increase, or improve the functional capabilities of individuals with disabilities, such as autism. An assistive technology service is any service that directly assists an individual with a disability in the selection, acquisition, or use of an assistive technology device. Generally, children with ASD process visual information easier than they do auditory information. Any time that you use assistive technology devices with your child, you are providing them with information through their strongest area of processing. Therefore, different forms of technology, for low to high-tech, can be integrated into most aspects of your child's daily life to improve their functional capabilities.

How Does Assistive Technology Help a Child With ASD?

The process of finding out the most effective assistive technology devices and services for your child begins with an evaluation. This can be conducted by an independent consultant or agency or the school that your child attends and should address both the challenges and strengths that your child possesses. Assistive technology is able to help your child learn their school material in a way that is easy for them to understand and can also break down the barriers they may face that prevent them from being at the same level as their peers and classmates.

As we have already stated, many children with ASD think visually – pictures are their first language, and words are their second. As literal, concrete, visuals thinkers, children with ASD can better process information when they are looking at images or words to help them visualize information. Technology simply makes visuals, like pictures, more accessible to a child with autism, and computer graphics can capture and maintain their attention. As we have already discussed in previous chapters, some children with autism may experience auditory sensitivities and are able to respond better to softer sounds.

Using computers, you can download appropriate voice levels and adjust the sound according to your child's needs.

There are plenty of applications out there that your child with autism, or you as their parent, can use that will automatically play a notification when the decibel level exceeds the set parameters.

Some individuals with ASD are incapable of sequencing. Technology can reduce the number of steps needed to complete a task, or can provide a visual representation of the sequence of steps required to complete a task. Moreover, individuals with autism will often experience difficulty with their fine motor skills, which can make writing difficult. Technology has the answer to this as well and can ease the frustration of handwriting or drawing using a keyboard, touchscreen, or speech-to-text to reduce frustration and difficulty, which subsequently increases the individual's enjoyment of learning.

For children with autism who do not use speech to communicate, they may need additional augmentation to produce verbal words and thoughts when faced with high-stress situations. Technology can aid in this and can be used as a voice output device to speak for them and help them fluently express themselves without ever needing to open their mouths. Nonspeaking children with autism generally find it easier to associate words with images if they are able to see the picture and its associated word printed together.

It is thought that some autistic individuals are incapable of listening and looking simultaneously. Their immature sensory system is not able to process visual and auditory input that occurs at the same time, but using technology, they can improve their ability to use both, or alternate between the two, gradually.

STRATEGIES FOR USING ASSISTIVE TECHNOLOGY FOR COMMUNICATION

The strategies that are used with assistive technology for communication can be placed into three different categories: high-tech strategies, mid-tech strategies, and low-tech strategies. Let's take a look at these categories.

High-Tech Strategies

These are the complex technical support strategies that generally involve 'high' cost equipment like computers, video cameras, and adaptive hardware, as well as complex voice output devices. Some of the skills that high-tech strategies are used to develop include social and language skills, and nonverbal cues like tone of voice, facial expressions, body language, etc., can be demonstrated and studied using videos. The use of computers by children with ASD can also increase their focus and attention while simultaneously improving their fine motor skills and reducing their agitation. In some cases, the computer will need to be adapted to meet the specific needs of the child, though this is generally not a challenge.

Mid-Tech Strategies

Mid-tech strategies involve some or other battery-powered device, like a Language master, tape recorder, timer, overhead projector, calculator, or simple voice output devices that enhance certain areas of skill. Most of the devices that fit into this category refer to Voice Output Communication Aids or VOCAs, and it is essential to understand that such devices were developed for use as an augmentative means to communicate expressively. Mid-tech strategies help develop skills that involve expressive communication, language comprehension, organization, social, and academic skills.

Low-Tech Strategies

These are the most affordable strategies. For instance, visual support strategies that do not involve any form of electronic technology, like clipboards, dry erase boards, manila file folders, laminated photographs, and so on. Consistent use of individualized schedules can help improve your child's organizational skills while simultaneously encouraging independence and reducing challenging behavior.

Examples of such schedules include things like visual routine checklists and calendars that tell a child exactly what is happening at the moment, what they can expect to happen next, and any changes that may take place. With the completion of each task, the child can make a mark on the schedule indicating that the task has been done. Be sure to use images that your child will find helpful – for instance, if colors tend to overstimulate or confuse your young one, rather use visuals in black and white.

GENERAL TIPS

Now that we've covered all of the basics when it comes to encouraging your child with autism to communicate with you and with others, we can move on to some general tips that you can implement to further foster communication. Once again, I must stress that not all children with autism are the same, and one strategy that may work for someone else's child with ASD may not work for yours, so be sure to try all of these to find one that does.

Make an Effort to Talk to Your Child

Since talking to a child with Autism Spectrum Disorder can be difficult, many parents simply take the easy way out and avoid including their child in conversations in the first place. Of course, this is a huge mistake – both you and your child can benefit from attempts at conversation, even if they are not always successful. There is also the tendency to assume that if a child with autism does not respond or shuts you down, they do not like you or do not want to talk to you. However, this is hardly ever the case – this signal would be crystal clear from a neurotypical child, but for someone with autism, it is just another part of the syndrome. Do not take it personally, and do not cease attempting to involve your child in your conversations, gently. Chances are, they really want to engage with you, but they just can't figure out how to.

Pick Your Moments

Not all times are the right times to talk to your child with ASD. Many children with autism will have very particular patterns and rhythms to their behavior, and if you interrupt them when they are wholly invested in something else, you are unlikely to be able to engage with them as much as you would have liked. Similarly, it is generally not a good idea to engage with your child when something else already has them wound up. Excessive stimuli can cause your ASD child to shut down. Wait for them to calm down, and once things are quiet, you can make another attempt at conversation.

Talk About What They Want to Talk About

One approach that is guaranteed to get you to know where when trying to talk to your child is trying to force the conversation in the direction that you want it to go. At best, you're going to get bored; at worst, your child will experience an outburst or will shut down. Obsessions are another part of the spectrum, and an obsession is going to mean plenty of discussion about one particular subject. While you may find it simple or boring, your child will find it the most interesting thing in the world, and you're going to get much more engagement out of them by sticking to the topic that they want to talk about.

Keep Things Concise and To the Point

As much as possible, try to stay away from metaphors, allusions, or any statements that can be considered abstract. Children on the spectrum will often not be able to understand any form of communication that relies on reading your internal emotional stage or any kind of subtext whatsoever. Thus, you should be keeping your sentences direct and short. The pace of the conversation should be one that your child is capable of maintaining. For most neurotypical individuals, processing sentences is a piece of cake and is something that we do as we hear them – it happens almost instantaneously. Children with autism need to work to decipher the things they hear, though, so you should give your child the time they need to do just that.

Observe Your Child's Nonspeaking Cues

Since children with ASD can experience difficulty understanding and manipulating language, they often develop many different forms of behaviors that represent things you may not have expected them to verbalize. Specific actions or motions that your child might use when talking may tell you more than the words they speak if you pay close attention and learn to interpret them.

Remember, your child is just that – a child. While they might not behave like a neurotypical child, remember that you are still talking to a person whose attitudes and thoughts are being formed in an immature brain. With some practice, you might find that you can talk to your child the same way you would with any other neurotypical child. The results, for both you and them, can be positive when it comes to their communication skill development, and enjoyable as you strengthen the bond between you two.

Chapter references

Applied Behavioral Analysis. (2017, December 1). *7 Tips for Talking to Kids with Autism.* Applied Behavioral Analysis | How to Become an Applied Behavior Analyst. https://www.appliedbehavioranalysisedu.org/7-tips-for-talking-to-kids-with-autism/

En, U. (n.d.). *ASSISTIVE TECHNOLOGY: A support for children with autism spectrum disorder.* Upbility EN. Retrieved February 21,

2021, from https://upbility.net/blogs/news/assistive-technology-a-support-for-children-with-autism-spectrum-disorder

Helping your child with nonspeaking autism talk. (2013, March 19). Autism Speaks. https://www.autismspeaks.org/expert-opinion/seven-ways-help-your-child-nonverbal-autism-speak

Miller, C. (2019, October 14). *Helping Children With Autism Learn to Communicate.* Child Mind Institute. https://childmind.org/article/helping-children-with-autism-learn-to-communicate/

5

TEACHING SOCIAL SKILLS TO YOUR CHILD WITH ASD

As we have already discussed numerous times throughout this book, children with autism struggle to understand and learn social skills and cues. It is one of the biggest challenges that they face, and it often leaves them isolated from their classmates and peers, as they feel like they are 'other'. Teaching your child social skills can help them understand how to act in various social situations, from playing with their friends at school to talking to their distant relatives. Social skills will help your ASD child make friends, develop their hobbies and interests, and learn from others. These skills are also able to help with family relationships. In essence, social skills will give your child that sense of belonging that they crave, which will improve their mental health and overall quality of life.

It will be highly beneficial for your child to develop play skills, such as sharing a toy or taking turns in a game; conversation skills, such as learning what body language to use and choosing what to talk about;

emotional skills, such as empathy and emotional management; and problem-solving skills, such as making decisions in a social situation and dealing with conflict. These skills will allow your child to engage in social interactions effortlessly and calmly, and they will also help them make new friends and maintain their friendships. One of the most important things to a child on the spectrum is a friend, and even if they make just one friend, they will be so much happier for it. In this chapter, we will discuss in more detail the reason that children with ASD suffer in social situations and what can be done to remedy this, as well as some useful strategies for teaching your child to interact with their classmates.

CHILDREN ON THE SPECTRUM STRUGGLE WITH SOCIAL SKILLS

Social dysfunction can manifest itself in a range of behaviors, from totally avoiding any kind of interpersonal interactions to completely monopolizing conversations on a sole topic that no one other than the individual talking seems to be interested in. There is no fixed pattern to social dysfunction, but it is almost always one of ASD's major identifiers. It is often the symptom that stands out the most when interacting with an individual on the spectrum. For ASD individuals who are high-functioning, social deficit skills can be so minor that they are nearly undetectable in casual conversation. These individuals generally develop coping mechanisms or are able to learn the skills needed to 'fit in' with their peers better. With proper training, which generally includes aspects of applied behavior analysis, they are generally capable of making a lot of progress in their social development. Nevertheless, at some level, even the highest-functioning autistic individuals almost always struggle with some ineptitude or discomfort in social situations.

On the other hand, those with low-functioning autism will generally display immediate and obvious struggles in social situations. However, they possess an advantage over their high-functioning counterparts in that they often experience less anxiety regarding their ineptitude in common social interactions due to their general inward focus. While they will also benefit from applied behavior analysis therapy to improve their social skills, they will always face the challenge of noticeable social deficits, and they will likely always find it almost impossible to naturally 'fit in' to common social situations.

What Is the Connection Between Autism & Social Skills?

Social skills are the customs, rules, and abilities that guide our interactions with the world and people around us. Generally, we tend to learn social skills in the same way we learn how to use language - easily and naturally. Over time, we create a social map of how to act in various situations with others. For people with autism, learning these skills does not come as naturally and requires some extra effort. The development process involves focusing on attention and timing, explicit instruction and 'teachable moments' with practice in realistic settings, a way to accumulate language and cognitive skills, support for the enhancement of communication and sensory integration, and learning behaviors that predict essential social outcomes, like happiness and friendship.

The inability to read nonverbal communication cues, difficulty and delays in acquiring verbal communication skills, overwhelming sensory inputs, obsessive or repetitive behaviors, and the insistence on sticking to a fixed routine are all problems with social skills that are rooted in some of ASD's basic elements. This combination of attributes makes it extremely challenging for children with ASD to develop the basic social skills that all neurotypical individuals take for granted. This deficiency is often misinterpreted as a desire to avoid social interactions or people, in general, but this could not be more untrue – the majority of autistic individuals crave interaction with others but simply lack the skills to do so effortlessly.

This leads to frustration that fuels itself. Individuals with ASD may throw tantrums, have outbursts, or express themselves in an inappropriate way in social contexts, which is a result of them boiling over at their own difficulty to either make themselves understood to others or to understand their own place in social situations. On the other hand, at the opposite end of the spectrum – though still completely rooted in deficits in social skills – some individuals cannot fully understand their own issues with communication and often fail to recognize how their means of communication may make others feel uncomfortable or offended. These sorts of social errors are due to obliviousness – being unwilling or unable to converse outside a particular topic, monopolizing conversations, or generally ignoring all external stimuli.

Who Can Teach Social Skills?

There are plenty of social skills to learn, so different people will teach them in different ways and in different settings – at school, at home, and throughout the community. A speech-language pathologist, special education teacher, or other clinician might lead a social skills group that combines explicit, direct instruction with opportunities to generalize and practice these skills in environments that are more natural. This means real-life practice with peers.

Social skills groups provide autistic individuals with the opportunity to practice their social skills with their neurotypical peers on a regular basis, no matter their age. Many groups follow commercially available social skills curricula, and a review of five studies regarding social skills groups by researchers at the University of Utah and the U.C. Davis MIND Institute helped identify what makes social skills groups effective. In essence, a social skills group should break down abstract social concepts into concrete actions, work in groups with encouraged partnership and cooperation, provide stability and structure, simplify language and group individuals by language level, foster self-awareness and esteem, and provide varied and multiple learning opportunities.

Teaching Social Skills

As a parent, it is understandable that you are probably eager to start teaching your child social skills right away, but there are a few steps that must be taken before this can happen. If you do not take these steps, then the education will likely be ineffective, and you and your child will only find yourself more frustrated. In this section, we'll discuss the steps you should take before teaching social skills and how you can actually begin teaching social skills.

ASSESSING SOCIAL FUNCTIONING

The first step in any training program for social skills should involve a thorough evaluation of your child's current level of social functioning. The goal for this evaluation is to answer one very simple, yet also complicated, question: *What is preventing your child from forming and maintaining social relationships?* For most children, the answer has to do with deficits in social skills, while for some, the answer has to do with the cruelty of their peers. Sometimes, the answer is both.

This evaluation should detail both the areas of strength and weakness of your child in relation to social functioning, and it should involve a combination of observation, interview, and standardized measures, like social skills measures and behavioral checklists. It is essential that your child's team of clinicians ascertains the child's current level of functioning and effectively intervenes at the determined area of need. For example, if the assessment reveals that your child is not capable of maintaining simple one-on-one interactions with others, then the process of intervention should start at this level, not at a more advanced level. Alternatively, if the assessment reveals that your child does not know how to play with items functionally or how to play symbolically, then the intervention should begin by teaching play skills *before* teaching specific interaction skills. After the thorough evaluation of social functioning is done, the team should determine whether the skill deficits are the result of performance deficits or skill acquisition deficits.

Acquisition Deficits vs. Performance Deficits

After you have completed the assessment of your child's social functioning, and after you have identified the skills that must be taught, you will need to determine whether the skills deficits are caused by acquisition deficits or performance deficits. In layman's terms, the success of the social skills training is dependent on your ability to make this distinction.

A skill acquisition deficit is the absence of a certain behavior or skill. For instance, a young child with autism might not know how to join activities with their peers effectively, which will often lead them to fail to participate. If we want this child to join peer activities, they must be taught the appropriate skills to do so.

On the other hand, a performance deficit is a behavior or skill that is present but is not performed. Using the same example, a child might possess the ability to join activities with their peers, but they fail to do so for whatever reason. In this case, if we want the child to interact with their peers, we do not need to teach them how. We must address the factor that is preventing them from doing so. This could be due to anxiety, a lack of motivation, or sensory over-sensitivities.

A good way to make the distinction between an acquisition and performance deficit is to ask, "Can my child do the task with several people in different settings?" For example, if your child only initiates interactions with you at home and not with their peers at school, then you should address the difficulty in initiation as a skill acquisition deficit. Often, a deficit in social skills and inappropriate behaviors are incorrectly identified as deficits in performance. That is, we want to assume that when a child is not performing a certain behavior, it is because they refuse to or are not motivated to.

The benefit of using the model of skill acquisition/performance deficit is that it guides the selection of intervention strategies. Most of these strategies are better suited for one of the two, but not both. Once the thorough assessment of social skills has been completed, and your child's team of clinicians can determine whether they are experiencing a performance or acquisition deficit, you can begin instruction in social skills. There are several strategies that you can use with your young one. Let's take a look at them.

Accommodation & Assimilation

When choosing a strategy for intervention, it is important to take into consideration the idea of accommodation versus assimilation. In the context of teaching social skills, accommodation involves the act of changing the social or physical environment of your child to encourage positive social interaction. Examples include autism awareness training for classmates and signing your child up for group activities, like Girl or Boy Scouts or little league sports.

On the other hand, assimilation involves helping your child grow and change. It involves teaching that fosters the development of social skills, which allows your child to be more successful in their social interactions. The trick to a successful social skills training program is to address both of these concepts. Only focusing on one will set your child up for failure. You can not provide your child with opportunities to interact with others without teaching them the skills they need for successful interactions, and vice versa. The key is to teach skills and modify the environment, ensuring that the new skills are received by your child's peers with acceptance and understanding.

Thoughts & Feelings Activities

Identifying and understanding the thoughts and feelings of oneself is often an area of weakness for children on the spectrum, but it is essential to successful social interactions. For example, we constantly modify our behavior based on the nonverbal feedback we receive from others. If another person is smiling, looking on intently, or showing other signs of interest, then we may elaborate on a story. Conversely, if they sigh or look otherwise disinterested, we might cut the story short. Children with ASD will experience difficulty identifying and understanding these unspoken cues, and it is because of this that they are less capable of altering their behavior to meet the cognitive and emotional needs of others.

The simplest thought and feeling activity consists of showing your child images of people displaying various emotions. These images can range from basic emotions, like sad, happy, scared, or angry, to more complex ones, like nervous, embarrassed, or confused. Start by asking your child to point to an emotion – "Point to *happy*" – then ask them to identify what the person in the image is feeling – "How is he feeling?"

Many young ASD children are actually capable of acquiring this ability quite seamlessly, and when they do, it will be time to progress to instructional strategies that are more advanced, like teaching them to understand the "why" behind emotions. To do this, the child must make inferences based on the cues and context that the picture provides. In essence, based on the information in the picture, you can ask, "why is the child sad?" The pictures will need to display people engaging in different social situations and portraying different facial expressions or other nonverbal emotional expressions.

Once your child has achieved mastery over these pictures, you can move on to video footage or TV programs of social situations. Children's networks are a great resource for this.

Peer-Mediated Interventions

Using peer mentors is one example of an effective strategy. Peer-mediated interventions (PMIs) have been used frequently to promote positive social interactions specifically amongst preschool-aged peers, and it allows you to structure the social and physical environment in a way that encourages successful social interactions. Using this strategy, peers are trained systematically to initiate interactions or respond appropriately and promptly to the initiations of the child with ASD throughout the duration of the school day. These peer mentors should be classmates of the child and have play and social skills appropriate to their age, as well as a regular attendance record and positive history of interactions with the child with ASD.

Peer mentors will need to be informed of the behaviors that are associated with ASD in a way that is developmentally appropriate and respectful for the age group. Using peer mentors allows the teacher and other adults to serve as facilitators rather than active participants. It also facilitates skill generalization by ensuring that newly acquired skills are practiced and performed with peers in a natural environment.

Behavioral Rehearsal / Role-Playing

This strategy is mainly used to teach basic social interaction skills. It is an effective approach to teaching skills that foster the positive practice of said skills. Role-playing involves acting out scenarios in a controlled environment to practice newly acquired skills or skills that were previously learned that the child is struggling to perform. Role-playing can be spontaneous or scripted. In the former scenario, the child is provided with a scenario, such as asking another child to play, but not with a predetermined script.

During the first couple of sessions, it is not unusual for a child to get 'stuck' in an interaction or conversation, often for a matter of minutes, without knowing how to proceed or what to say. During the early sessions, the child should be given plenty of time to process and respond to the scenarios, and as the sessions move on, proficiency and speed should progress, as well.

Implementing Intervention

After you have evaluated social skill functioning, identified skills to teach, distinguished between skill performance and acquisition deficits, and selected strategies for intervention, it is time to implement those strategies. Instruction on social skills should be offered in a number of settings and by numerous providers. There is no 'best' place for social skills to be taught, though it is important to remember that the purpose of all social skills instruction is to promote social success with peers in a natural environment. Thus, if your child is receiving social skills training from a private therapist or in a school resource room, it is vital that a plan be made to promote the transfer of skills from the isolated area to a natural environment. You should look for opportunities to reinforce and prompt the skills that your child is being taught.

I have said it before, and I will say it again - every child on the spectrum is different, and the rate at which your child develops their social skills will differ greatly from another child. Some may start to use their skills after just a few sessions, while others may need months of training before they get it. Simply trying to use a social skill is the first step that your child must take toward their social success. They can take all of the extra time they need to master the social skills that they are developing.

Assessing & Altering Instruction

While this may be the last stage in the process of intervention, it is not any less important. It is also not the last thing you should think about when designing a social skills training regimen. If possible, as soon as you have been able to identify the social skill problem areas that need to be addressed, you should try to develop methods for assessing the intervention's efficacy. For instance, if the goal is to teach your child how to initiate social interactions, then you should determine how often your child is doing so. Accurately collecting this information will allow you to determine if your child is benefitting from the intervention and how you should alter the training to meet their needs.

In a school setting, the accurate collection of data is a matter of legality. It needs to happen.

More About Strategies

As we mentioned above, social skills must generally be explicitly taught to children and adolescents with ASD. Traditional social skills strategies, like board games about friendship, are often too subtle for children with ASD to understand. There are many essential questions to ask when choosing an appropriate social skills strategy. Does the strategy target the skill deficits identified in the social assessment? Does the strategy encourage skill acquisition? Does the strategy enhance performance? Does research support its use?

BACK TO SCHOOL TIPS

The beginning of each new school year is both an exciting and anxious time for both parents and children, especially when it comes to children with ASD. It typically brings about change to the daily routine that was established during the summer, and the transition can be especially hard on children with autism. While this change can be difficult, there are a number of things you can do to prepare your child to take on the new school year and make the back-to-school transition an easy one.

Here are some tips and tricks:

Prepare and reintroduce routines - The first thing you should do is familiarize and reintroduce your child to the school setting. This might involve showing your child a picture of their teacher and some of their classmates or bringing them to the classroom to get them familiar with the environment and faces that they can expect to see once again. If you can, try to arrange to visit your child's teacher a week or two before the first day back, but if you are not able to do this, you could opt to spend some time on the playground or visit the school building.

Driving past the school a few times can also help, and you may want to drive your child to school on their first day. For many children with ASD, taking the bus to school on the very first day can trigger a sensory overload. Steadily easing them into the routine of transportation will be helpful for everyone involved.

Teach and review social expectations - While many children might find the transition between the social demands of summer activities and those needed in the classroom easy, children on the spectrum may need clearer, more literal reminders. Be sure to review what behavior is acceptable at school and what behavior is not. You could also create a schedule of a typical day at school using images and talk about how days at school will progress – create a picture schedule or social story for school routines.

It helps to start reviewing, practicing early, and if possible, meeting with teachers and admins to discuss your child's unique strengths and difficulties. Remember that you are the best advocate for your child, even if you have hired a professional. Communication should be established early on to foster positive relationships with your child's school and their teachers. Rehearse new activities and ask your child's teacher what new activities are planned for the first week of school. Then, prepare your child by practicing, performing, and discussing them – this rehearsal will help ease anxiety when new activities happen during the start of school.

Expect the unexpected - It is impossible for you as a parent to predict every single thing that may happen in a school day. Allocate more time for all activities throughout the first week back, and prepare your child for scenarios that might not go as planned. Again, use social stories to familiarize your child with routines and how to respond when an unexpected occurrence...occurs. The noise, activity, and chaos of a typical classroom and cafeteria can sometimes be overwhelming, so expect and prepare for sensory overload. Concoct a plan for this situation, finding out if there might be a quiet room in the school where your child can take a quick break.

Cross days off of the calendar - If your child is experiencing anxiety when the school year starts, simply crossing days off of the calendar can help them understand when school starts, thus easing their anxiety.

Develop a new morning routine and practice it before school starts - Start waking your child up a bit earlier every morning so that they grow used to the new wake-up time before the first day. Do a couple of run-throughs near the end of vacation so that they know what to expect in the time before leaving for school. If your child is responsive to visual schedules, you can develop one that outlines everything that happens on a school day, from getting dressed in the morning to getting on the bus.

Tour the school - You can arrange this with the case manager for your child's study team. You might not be able to meet your child's new teacher before the first day, but they will at least be able to familiarize themselves with the school building before it becomes crowded with children and teachers. When on the tour, be sure to stop at the main office, cafeteria, bathrooms, playground, library, and any other room that your child may find themselves in throughout the year. Take a few photographs on the tour and include them in a social story afterward so that you can review it with your child during the summer.

Practice emergency procedures - This is a particularly important step if your child experiences sensory overload. If possible while on your tour, ask your case manager to show your child what to do and where to go during an emergency scenario. Doing so will help prepare them, and they might even find it fun to have you practice while standing next to them silently.

Write a letter detailing the needs of your child - If you can, have your young one help you create this document since it will provide valuable input for the staff at school. Ensure that you include a few things that are unique and fun about your child, and a copy of this letter (two pages maximum) should go to your child's teacher and aides. It should also be available to any and all staff that work with them. Remember to send a copy to the principal, vice principal, physical therapist, occupational therapist, PE teacher, speech therapist, music teacher, and so on. It is extremely helpful for teachers to have a 'glimpse' at your child before interacting with them. Don't be afraid to brag, either!

Augmentative devices - If your child uses an augmentative device to aid in communication, make sure that all of the adults in their classroom are familiar with it. Many of these devices require some instruction regarding their use, and at the very least, your child's teacher should be familiar with them before school starts. All of the aides that work with your child should be familiar with it, as well, and there should also be a plan in place so that everyone can use it comfortably within the first couple of weeks after school starts.

Meet the bus driver - Many bus drivers will do a practice run the week before school starts. Request a meeting with them so that your child can be introduced and feel comfortable riding the bus the first time they are on it. You can even ask if your child can ride with the driver on their practice run.

TIPS FOR TEACHERS

If you happen to be a teacher reading this, then you may want to learn more about how you can improve the school life of an autistic student. If you are a parent, then you can pass the following tips on to your child's teacher.

Learn About the Student From the Student

Educators who need information about a student will often study their educational records, and while these documents are definitely a source of information, they are rarely the most useful source. Teachers who want to know more about a student with autism should ask the student to provide that information. Some will be more than happy and able to share about themselves, while others might need coaxing or family support. If the student cannot communicate reliably, then teachers should turn to the family for help. Parents can share teaching tips that they found the most helpful at home, or they can share a video of the student participating in various family and community activities.

Teach To Interests

When possible, teachers should use strengths, interests, areas of expertise, skills, and gifts as teaching tools. Try to turn an autistic student's interests into a teaching opportunity, as it will help keep them engaged and actually make them enthusiastic about learning new material.

Get the Student Talking

In many classrooms, a small group of learners dominates small-group conversations and class-wide discussions. While it is important for these outgoing and verbal learners to have a voice, it is just as important for other learners, including those with disabilities, to have opportunities to challenge and share ideas, answer and ask questions, and vocalize their thoughts. Teachers should put up activities and structures that encourage interaction to ensure that all students are given the opportunity to communicate.

Teachers are also able to encourage communication by giving every student the chance to talk during a class discussion. Instead of asking, "Who can tell me a fraction that equals half?", a teacher could say, "Stand up if you think you can name a fraction that equals half." Not only does this strategy give all learners a chance to answer the question, but it also allows for some movement, which is often treasured by students with ASD.

Provide Choices

Not only can choice allow students to feel as if they are in control of their lives, but it also provides them with an opportunity to discover themselves more as learners and workers. Choice can be particularly useful for students with ASD who have certain needs concerning lesson materials, learning environment, and communication. Choice can be incorporated into almost any part of the school day. Learners can choose which role to take in a collaborative group, which assessments to complete, and how to receive support and personal assistance.

Create a Comfortable Classroom

Students are sometimes unsuccessful as a result of discomfort or fear they feel in their educational environment. Ensuring that a learning environment is appropriate is as essential to the success of students as any educational tool or teaching strategy. Students with ASD will be the most willing to learn in places where they can feel secure and relaxed. To make the classroom more comfortable, teachers can include various seating options like bean bag chairs, reducing direct light where possible, and minimizing distracting noises.

You're almost at the end! In the next and final chapter, we'll discuss how to teach your family about autism and how to interact with your child.

Chapter references

17 tips to help the transition back to school for kids with autism. (2018, July 7). Autism Speaks. https://www.autismspeaks.org/blog/17-tips-help-transition-back-school-kids-autism

Applied Behavioral Analysis. (2017, December 1). *Why Do Autistics Have Issues with Social Skills?* Applied Behavioral Analysis | How to Become an Applied Behavior Analyst. https://www.appliedbehavioranalysisedu.org/why-do-autistics-have-issues-with-social-skills/

Bellini, S. A. D. (n.d.). *Making (and Keeping) Friends: A Model for Social Skills Instruction.* Indiana Resource Center for Autism. Retrieved February 23, 2021, from https://www.iidc.indiana.edu/irca/articles/making-and-keeping-friends.html

Kluth, P. (2019, December 18). *Supporting Students with Autism: 10 Ideas for Inclusive Classrooms.* Reading Rockets. https://www.readingrockets.org/article/supporting-students-autism-10-ideas-inclusive-classrooms

Social skills for children with autism spectrum disorder. (2020, May 13). Raising Children Network. https://raisingchildren.net.au/autism/communicating-relationships/connecting/social-skills-for-children-with-asd

Wilkinson, L. A. (2020, March 2). *Back to School - tips for parents of children on the autism spectrum.* Living Autism. https://livingautism.com/back-school-tips-parents-children-autism-spectrum/

6

ASD & FAMILY COMMUNICATION

Throughout this book, we have discussed the challenges that children with ASD face, as well as their strengths, weaknesses, and unique needs. By now, you should know just about everything you would need to know about autism as a parent, but it doesn't stop there. If you are a parent of multiple children, both neurotypical and autistic, then you likely want to know how to teach your neurotypical children about autism and about how they should interact with their autistic sibling. This is a common concern amongst parents, as neurotypical children might not understand why their autistic sibling is different from the other children at school.

If you were raised with siblings, then you have likely been influenced by that relationship. However, living with an autistic sibling adds more unique and significant experiences to that relationship – when one child in the family has a disability, it affects the entire family. Every member of the family can be both stressed and strengthened by this situation, though there are some tips that I can provide to strengthen your family bond and minimize stressors.

While an autism diagnosis can challenge the unique relationship between siblings, all siblings can learn from one another, have meaningful and positive relationships, and bring out the best in each other. As with any family, there will be aspects of family life that are going to be trying. However, most children are able to handle challenges well, especially when they receive support and understanding from their parents. The content in this chapter not only applies to siblings but to distant relatives, as well, such as cousins.

HELPING SIBLINGS OF CHILDREN WITH AUTISM SPECTRUM DISORDER

Your child's siblings are some of the most important people in their life, especially if they are of similar ages. Siblings can be a great source of support for your child who is on the spectrum and can promote their development in ways you may have never imagined. In this section, I will give you some tips that you can pass on to your neurotypical children to help them interact with their autistic sibling and support them.

Teach neurotypical siblings to be proud of your child with ASD – Teach your children how to talk about autism and how to be comfortable describing the disorder to others. If they are comfortable with the topic, your ASD child will be more comfortable, as well. If they are too embarrassed by their sibling, their friends will pick up on that and make things awkward for everyone. If a neurotypical sibling is able to talk openly to their friends about autism, they will not only make their autistic sibling more comfortable overall, but they will also share their knowledge with their friends and make their friends more understanding.

Remind them that some sadness is natural – It is completely normal for neurotypical children to feel a little sad that their sibling is affected by autism, but you should remind them that getting upset will not help anybody and will likely only make things more difficult. Remind them that you also feel sad sometimes but that you have to work together to push through it and make life better for the whole family.

Spend time with neurotypical children – Getting wrapped up in the wellbeing and care of your child with ASD happens very quickly, and it can take a while for you to realize that you have not been paying your neurotypical children the same amount of attention. You should not feel guilty about this – children with ASD require more special attention than their neurotypical siblings – but try to spend some alone time with your neurotypical children, as well, perhaps when your child with ASD is taking a nap.

Find activities that the whole family can do together – Neurotypical children will find it rewarding to bond with their autistic sibling, even if the activity is just putting together a simple puzzle. Regardless of your child with ASD's level of functioning, doing something together fosters closeness. They will always look forward to spending time with their siblings, and vice versa.

YOUR NEUROTYPICAL CHILDREN SHOULD KNOW WHAT AUTISM IS

Be sure to explain autism to your neurotypical children using concepts and words that are appropriate for their age and understanding. Learning about the condition will help siblings better understand their autistic sibling and why they require special attention from their parents. Talking to a sibling about autism is also not going to be a once-off conversation but rather a dialogue that will continue to grow over time. Often, siblings of children on the spectrum gain a unique insight into the family situation, and as a parent, it is important for you to listen to what your neurotypical children are trying to tell you.

Set the stage early for honest and open communication so that all of your children feel comfortable expressing concerns and frustrations or asking questions. If you do this, you might hear from siblings that they do not know how to connect to their autistic sibling, are concerned about their privacy, wish they could spend some more time with you alone, have become the target of aggressive behavior, are feeling stressed about increased responsibility, and worry about their parents or the future. These are all normal concerns, and it is important for siblings to know that you are there to listen to them and take care of them.

Remember that the special bond that forms between neurotypical siblings can also exist with siblings with autism. You may find that your child is more verbal or social with their neurotypical sibling than they are with anyone else. Siblings, especially when young, can be very creative in finding ways to interact and play with their autistic sibling, so you should allow the space for them to get to know each other and enjoy each other's company.

TEACHING SIBLINGS ABOUT AUTISM SPECTRUM DISORDER

Dealing with neurotypical siblings is already a challenge in the best of circumstances, but when one of them is autistic, the challenges multiply. How do you deal with it, then? The best way is to teach your children what ASD is. You will be able to help them deal with the confusion and complexity that sharing a childhood with a sibling on the spectrum entails, which will also help strengthen their bonds.

Explaining without labels – You could define autism as a disorder and explain it on those terms, or you can look at it as a different aspect of what some think of as 'normal'. Both of these things include the use of labels. While labels can help us order and categorize our lives, they can also stigmatize, hurt, and confuse us. Of course, the word autism is a label, and we use it to communicate certain information with a child's teacher, doctor, or caregiver. When you use that label with one of your neurotypical children, depending on how old they are, it may not be helpful. A five-year-old, for instance, will not understand why their eight-year-old sibling bangs their head and screams by simply learning that their sibling has autism.

Labels also tend to lead to a feeling of separation that can work against your best efforts of fostering a closer family unit in which siblings are genuinely compassionate and understanding toward their sibling with ASD. Try explaining the condition in terms that invoke a sense of familial compassion and duty to look after the autistic sibling. This will give your neurotypical children a sense of inclusion and belonging that comes from having an important role as a protector and guardian. You are going to have to find other words to help gain understanding in the context of how your family views autism as a condition. How you do that and what you believe is best for your family is up to you.

Always be honest – It is important to talk to your neurotypical children about how their sibling's condition will affect them. At every stage of development, new challenges will present themselves, and there is no way to avoid the fact that these challenges will have an impact on everyone in the family in one way or another. The older your child with autism becomes, the more aware they will become of how different they are from the rest of the family depending, of course, on where your child is on the spectrum.

Thus, when it comes to a family with an autistic member, honestly truly is the best policy. You should not restrain yourself from letting your children know when you are feeling frustrated, as this type of honesty will encourage your neurotypical children to be honest, as well. This will, in turn, give them power over their negative emotions. Honest communication will also provide your children with the freedom to ask questions that might be considered rude, inappropriate, or inconsiderate in other circumstances. Your children need answers just as much as you do, and while they might ask different questions or have different feelings, they are legitimate.

Acknowledging their emotions and questions will help them understand and cope.

Join an autism support group – Your children will sometimes need to hear it from someone else. Raising a child on the spectrum will challenge even the most prepared and resilient parents, and the same goes for your neurotypical children. They will experience things that will change their lives and often make them more difficult. Support groups for families with autism can be a fantastic aid, as they will not only allow you and your family to share stories and experiences, but you may also be able to learn some tips from parents who are further down the road and who can offer wisdom based on their experiences.

Your neurotypical children will also get to spend time with other siblings of children with autism. Hearing from someone their age about how they feel frustrated or embarrassed can relieve feelings of anger and guilt in your child. It can also help them feel less alone to know that there are other children out there who share some of their experiences.

Let books do some of the explaining – The way that you talk to your neurotypical children will, of course, depend on their age. If you have a teen and decide later in life that you want another child, and that child is born with ASD, then your talk with your teenager about their new little sibling will be different than with a five-year-old. Books on autism – such as this one! – can be fantastic tools for helping younger children understand why their sibling is different.

Reading an age-appropriate book, then discussing it afterward with your child, will give them the chance to conceptualize the issue of autism in the abstract and also ask questions, which will foster empathy in them. Your child may not instantly empathize with their autistic sibling, but they will feel empathy for their favorite character in the book, which will translate to how they act and feel in the real world.

The discussion should be ongoing – Although there might be a key point in time when you sit your neurotypical children down to explain autism to them, the conversation will only have just begun. Every day brings out unique interactions between your child and their neurotypical siblings, and you will need to talk about what is going on to foster understanding. If you are constantly isolating your child with autism or are shielding your neurotypical children from things, you are building feelings of confusion and separation within the family unit.

Talking to your neurotypical children about their sibling with ASD is naturally going to be challenging, which is why you should rely on some outside assistance. This could mean finding a documentary or book on the subject or reaching out for help from others. Know that you are not alone, and there are many resources at your disposal to help make the discussion easier for both you and your children.

CHALLENGES & FEELINGS

As we have already discussed, growing up with a sibling with ASD presents a number of challenges that can lead to mixed emotions. Let's take a look at some of the challenges your neurotypical children might be facing and how you can help deal with them.

Negative Emotions

Autism presents a plethora of feelings that can be difficult for the whole family to process. Your children might face resentment, anger, loss, guilt, and many more feelings. They may not know how to cope or might not want to talk to you about their feelings for fear of sounding negative about their autistic sibling or seeming like a burden. This is why it is essential for you to assure your children that these feelings are natural. Listen to what they have to say, acknowledge their feelings as legitimate, and offer them suggestions on how to work through them.

Even if what they are saying is harsh, like "I hate my sister!", you will need to be open to these very real feelings as a parent and guide your children through the process of dealing with them. It is essential to maintain an open line of communication between you and your neurotypical children. You might want to present opportunities for discussion by revealing your own feelings and struggles in ways that your children will be able to understand and appreciate. Siblings of children on the spectrum sometimes feel more comfortable expressing themselves if they know that you are experiencing similar emotions. You should also remind your children that all siblings have moments where they do not get along or where they fight.

Encourage your neurotypical children to accept the challenges and responsibilities that come with being a sibling of someone with autism, but also remind them to appreciate the quirks that their sibling has. Everyone is different, and every person has something about them that can be appreciated. Your children will learn that better than most.

Thinking of the Future

As your children grow older and start to ponder their futures, they might ask you questions regarding where their autistic sibling fits in. When you feel that the time is right, be sure to involve them in the planning process. Once again, keeping an open line of communication will ensure that everyone is comfortable with any plans that have been put in place. If you will be unable to care for your child with autism preventatively, earlier discussions will help your neurotypical children deal with these kinds of situations as they present themselves.

If your child with ASD will require care in the future, it is important that you take the thoughts of your other children regarding the matter into consideration. You will likely find that your children develop a sense of responsibility for their autistic sibling at a young age, though some siblings might not have given the matter much thought. As a parent, the best thing you can do for your children is to be supportive of their decisions and validate their feelings regarding their autistic sibling in the future. One of your children might feel obliged to take responsibility, and they might also feel guilty if they do not feel confident enough in their desire or ability to do so.

Whatever decision your children make, your reassurance and guidance will allow them to feel more comfortable about the uncertainty of the future.

Aggressive Behaviors

When we were young, we were taught the basics of violence - hitting others is bad, and violence in any form is unacceptable. However, when a sibling with ASD is aggressive, the line becomes blurred. Violent tendencies are not always a symptom of autism, but they usually become a source of fear, tension, and stress within families. Your neurotypical children might ask you why their sibling gets away with being aggressive, and they may feel confused, upset, or even fearful if they see their autistic sibling hurting a family member or themselves. Some children might resent these violent outbursts or feel protective of parents that are the target of aggression.

Explaining the violent behavior of an autistic sibling is a sensitive process that should be delicately approached. Children on the spectrum can act out violently because they are in pain, experiencing sensory overload, or because they are frustrated. It can be worthwhile to explain to your neurotypical children that, while they can let someone know when they have been hurt or are bothered, it is not as simple for their autistic sibling to express themselves. You might feel tempted to say something like, "Your sibling can't help their behavior," Remember that this might make your other children feel unsupported or that their safety is not a priority.

You can soothe concerns and fears via a combination of comfort, explanations, and prevention plans. No matter what, the issue of violence must be addressed.

Strengthening the Sibling Relationship

Something that every parent wants is for their children to get along with one another, but this is a luxury that many parents of neurotypical children take for granted. It can sometimes be more difficult for siblings to bond when one is autistic, so here are a few tips you can implement to encourage bonding between your children.

Encourage time together and apart – For your neurotypical children, spending time with their autistic sibling can sometimes feel more like a chore than an activity to be enjoyed, particularly due to potential barriers like lack of communication, common interests, and displayed affection. This can make bonding an uphill battle, and unfortunately, children do not have the foresight to see the long-term benefits of fighting it. Frustration can be heightened if your child feels as though they are being forced to prioritize their autistic sibling over their friends because you are trying to force the relationship to prosper. The sibling relationship will be much healthier if your neurotypical children are given the time they need to spend with their friends.

Your neurotypical children will feel more inclined to spend time with their autistic sibling if they have other friends that they can do things with, like engaging in hobbies, enjoying common interests, and interacting socially. They will have gained the enjoyment from their friends that we as social humans need to feel fulfilled and happy. With this fundamental desire satisfied, your child will then have the motivation to enjoy themselves in other ways and form a different kind of friendship with their autistic sibling. It will be gratifying enough for them just to make their ASD sibling happy.

Emphasize your neurotypical child's role – Children enjoy feeling valued and wanted, and they enjoy feeling as though they are important and responsible. It is part of a natural craving for attention in a non-selfish way – everyone likes to be focused on every now and then. You can use this to prompt your neurotypical children to interact with their autistic siblings on their own terms, which will be much more effective than forcing them to play together. Praise your children for the role that they fulfill. Say things like, "You're super helpful! You read that book with your brother so well," or, "I love that you're such a good listener with your sister when she tells you about her new toys!"

This kind of positive reinforcement will convey valuable roles, and acknowledging that your neurotypical children are being helpful will make them feel more wanted and valued. Your children will also learn that interacting with their autistic sibling is an opportunity for them to feel proud and accomplished, and eventually, they will not play together because you asked them to but because they want to. This is essential for making children feel eager to do something.

Take your children on a playdate where other children will attend – At some stage, you will likely take your child on playdates with other children on the spectrum. Despite your best intentions, this might cause your neurotypical children to feel jealous, as they will not fully be able to understand that your child needs extra socialization. To them, it may appear that you favor one child over the other, so taking all of your children to a playdate will not only make your neurotypical children feel more included and reduce their jealousy, but it will also make your child with autism feel included.

More importantly, your neurotypical children might see other children with ASD with their neurotypical siblings and understand how the playdate is beneficial to everyone, which will bolster their understanding of the disorder. Additionally, attending a playdate that features both autistic and neurotypical families is a great way for your children to bond with others and relay feelings about their similar lives. This will help them understand that there are other families like yours out there that have the same challenges and experiences that they do.

Have one-on-one time – You should make time to go places and do things with your neurotypical children alone. If you have a partner, then they can stay with your ASD child while you spend some quality time with the others, and you both can take turns doing this. If you are a single parent, then you can always hire a babysitter to care for your child on the spectrum, but make sure that they are properly trained to care for a child on the spectrum.

You should also aim to give your neurotypical children one-on-one time every day, even if it is just for half an hour a few times a day. Whether it is something grander, like going to the pool or the fair for the day, or something small like taking them shopping or watching an episode of their favorite show with them, the individual, undivided attention will go a long way in making them feel loved, which will foster stronger bonds.

ADULT SIBLINGS

Being the sibling of an individual with Autism Spectrum Disorder does not end with childhood. It is a lifetime relationship that grows and matures over the years, and the concerns of an adult sibling will, of course, be different from those of a child. For the young adult, the questions they ask you may focus more on their own plans to have children, and they may ponder the concern about whether there is a genetic factor playing into their sibling's autism. In some cases, young adults can also feel that they have a responsibility for their autistic sibling, which can make it challenging for them to leave home and start their own independent lives.

You need to discuss with your adult children the expectations they have in caring for your child with autism, and also reassure them about the legitimacy of them assuming their own role as adults. The question of the role of the adult child becomes most prevalent as parents grow older and start to expect the point at which they will no longer be capable of caring for their child with ASD. If the child has not already moved away from home, this may be the time when placement in a supervised apartment or group home becomes viable. In families where this kind of care is necessary, adult children and their parents need to address the question of who will become the guardian of the child with autism when the parents have both passed away.

It is not easy to talk about our own deaths, and both you and your children might shy away from the conversation. Still, your adult children must understand the financial plans you have made, the care arrangements in place, and what you expect of them. Having these challenging conversations will, in the end, be a gift to your adult children, who know they can honor your wishes.

EXTENDED FAMILY & FRIENDS

Getting your extended family members and your friends to come to terms with the fact that your child is on the autism spectrum can be difficult at times. Some will deny that the child is even autistic at all, saying things like, "You just need to be a little more strict." Your extended family will only be able to help to the extent that they accept the diagnosis and actively support you. Sometimes, grandparents, aunts, and uncles will not accept your guidance and will offer treats or forbidden foods to your child. If this happens, you might need to limit contact between your child and them until they can properly understand your position on your child's treatment.

Sometimes, you will not receive any support at all from those you would expect it from, regardless of how much you want or need it. Other times, support will come from the people that you least expected it to come from. Remember that not every single member of your extended family needs to know that your child has autism, particularly if you rarely see them in the first place.

SECURITY & SAFETY

In any home where young children are growing up, added safety measures will be necessary. Children with ASD, however, will need safety measures for longer periods of time than their neurotypical counterparts – possibly for their entire lives. You will also need to fully understand that children on the spectrum sometimes participate in behaviors that are not only a danger to themselves but to those around them. You should become able to deal with your child's curiosity, like taking things apart.

To make your home a safer place for your child on the spectrum, use locks and child-proof electric outlet covers, rearrange any furniture that could be dangerous to your child, and make use of child safety gates to restrict certain areas of the home that would be too dangerous for your child.

ACTIVITIES & HOBBIES THE WHOLE FAMILY CAN ENJOY

To end on a positive note, let's take a look at some fun activities that you can enjoy with your entire family, autistic or otherwise. It can be easy to avoid trying new things with your family due to your child's possible sensory issues. However, the fact that individuals on the spectrum, especially children, might not ask for company or to explore new possibilities on their own does not mean you should give up. Rather, it is an opportunity for you to find the best way to reach out and learn from and with them.

Choosing the Right Activity

There are plenty of ways for you, your family, and your young one to enjoy various activities and hobbies together. In some cases, accommodations will be needed, but most of the time, autism is either a non-issue or actually serves as an advantage. However, the key to success is to choose an activity and a place that is comfortable for your child with ASD and that they will find interesting. To choose an appropriate activity, start by paying attention to your child at play, and if they are verbal, ask them questions. What do they enjoy, and how do they choose to share their interests with you?

Next, you should try joining your child's activity. Instead of jumping in with your own directions and ideas, follow their lead. Most of us have been taught that there is a right and a wrong way to build a structure or play a game, and we all want our children to do it 'the right way', but you are working with a child on the spectrum, and they are not bound by the same trivial rules that we are. The first and most crucial step involves communication and engagement, not instruction. Think of ways to develop your child's interest. How can you play an interactive role in their preferred pastimes? How are you able to expand their interests and help them explore their environment?

Take things one step at a time. Your child might love baseball cards, which is a fantastic interest to share, but that does not mean that they will enjoy an entire day at a major league game. Start slow, maybe by watching just one inning at a high school game. If there are challenges, think about ways to work around them to help your child cope.

The most important thing to do is have fun. The whole point of enjoying activities with your child is to build connections and enjoy yourselves, and don't forget to include your neurotypical children, as well, if you have any. If the experience becomes stressful for anyone, back off a bit and find a way to make things fun.

Here are some of the best activities to include.

Video Games

As you may already know, video games are not just for children, and they vary in their complexity and difficulty. Your child with autism might enjoy playing Minecraft or Stardew Valley all alone, but that doesn't mean you and your family can't join in on the fun. Rather than assuming you are not welcome, or that the games will be too difficult for you, take some time to ask questions, get the hang of the game, and get involved. If your child has just started their new game or is struggling with a more complicated one, then there's nothing wrong with playing something very simple.

Legos

Legos are more than just colorful plastic blocks, and they can actually be transformed into a full-scale, international scientific and artistic medium. If your child is a fan of Legos, you have an unlimited number of options at your disposal. Build from diagrams and blueprints or create your own cities. Watch The Lego Movie and go to Lego conventions. Get involved with Lego Mindstorms, then join clubs and go to competitions. Even take a trip to a Lego art show. There are endless possibilities, and all of them are amazing.

Cartoons & Anime

Cartoons are generally a favorite amongst those on the spectrum, and a surprising amount of autistic individuals love anime – a complex and beloved form of Japanese animation. The world of anime is enormous, and it's everywhere. Join your child in watching their favorite show, and you may even end up becoming a fan of the fantastical animation and bizarre storylines.

Fantasy & Science Fiction

Fantasy and science fiction are often highly interesting to individuals with autism, as they offer a way to immerse oneself in a completely foreign and fantastical world with its own rules and laws that are, frankly, much more interesting than our own. Depending on your child's abilities and level of interest, they may learn every detail of a certain fictional world, write their own stories, watch and rewatch films, attend conventions, read comics, or even create their own costumes. There is a whole world of opportunity for hobbyists waiting to be discovered.

Hiking or Walking

This is a particularly fun family activity, especially if your family enjoys spending time outdoors. People, especially children, with autism are rarely good at team sports, but many have a large pool of stamina and physical energy. If your child matches that description, then you should consider getting into hiking and walking. In some areas, hiking involves climbing a mountain, while in others, it means walking down a street. Regardless, it is a fantastic opportunity for your family to spend time together and get some exercise. You may even want to bring a pair of binoculars with you to do some trainspotting, bird watching, or star gazing if you plan on camping.

7

THE IMPORTANCE OF SEEKING AN ADVOCATE FOR YOUR CHILD

One of the most important things you can do as a parent of a child with autism is to work with your school district to ensure that they receive a proper, appropriate education, though this is generally easier said than done. Parents often feel as though they are not equal members of their child's educational team and that decisions are being made without their child's unique needs in mind.

Once you add on the complexities of special education laws, with procedures and timelines that most parents will find unfamiliar at best and baffling at worst, things can quickly become overwhelming for the majority of families. This is why seeking out the assistance of an advocate is essential.

Advocates can be 'employed' to make these situations and meetings more manageable and less stressful by encouraging, assisting, and educating your family in understanding the ramifications of your decisions. The right advocate for your family can have a lasting impact on everyone involved, including the staff of professionals supporting your child, your family, and ultimately, your child. This can be a positive or negative impact, and an advocate is not someone you choose without careful thought and discussion.

Advocacy services are organizations that provide independent advocates, but a parent or family member, social worker, teacher, or carer can act as an advocate as well. Choosing the wrong advocate can have a significant, lasting impact on the relationship between the agency and the family. Just as finding the right therapist, doctor, or teacher takes investigation and time, so too does obtaining an autism advocate for your child.

WHAT IS AN AUTISM ADVOCATE, AND WHAT DO THEY DO?

According to the definition in the 1999 Webster's New College Dictionary, *advocate* means 'to speak in favor of, one who supports a cause, or one who speaks on another's behalf'. An autism advocate, by this definition, is someone that will represent, speak on behalf of, and support your child in many of their endeavors, primarily in the classroom and their educational institution. They will fill a number of functions and roles when supporting you and your child with autism.

As a parent, you have a deep care for how your child grows and learns and about being an equal member of the team that oversees and develops or carries out your child's Individualized Education Program, or IEP. If you are not already aware, an IEP is a written document that is developed for each child attending a public school that is eligible for special education and is created through a team effort and reviewed at least once annually. Before an IEP can be compiled, your child must be eligible for special education.

A good advocate will want to help you take on a primary role in your child's education. They will not make decisions on your behalf or without your knowledge but will help you stay informed and help you consider alternatives and options. In other words, a good advocate will be an empowering force when working with you. Of course, not all advocates are the same, and the exact role that they play in your family and the education of your child will vary depending on their training, areas of expertise, experience, and personality, as well as the particular situation you are in.

Generally, an autism advocate will be able to answer your questions and simplify the tricky maze of education to move toward an education for your child that is effective and appropriate. They will examine your child's school records and test results to determine whether further assessment must be conducted and suggest possible educational or clinical areas to explore based on your child's unique needs.

Your advocate should be able to provide you with referrals to proven professionals, like valuators, physicians, speech therapists, educational consultants, physical therapists, and occupational therapists. They will be able to prepare the necessary documentation to support the program that your child needs, which will save you from the burden of having to organize these things yourself. An advocate will also aid you in the process from evaluation through eligibility and the development of your child's IEP.

Suggesting accommodations to add to your child's IEP to support their learning further is another crucial skill that you should look for in an autism advocate. They should be capable of monitoring your child's progress and requesting modifications to their programs as needed to curate the best educational experience possible for your child. Advocates should also explore and investigate alternative educational placements for your child, should their current one fail to meet their unique needs.

Because your autism advocate is familiar with local resources and practices, they will often see solutions that are not immediately obvious, at least not to you, which can be extremely useful for those times when you feel that you're all out of options. They will support you through mediation and other avenues for resolving disputes, relieving unnecessary stress. While most are not attorneys, skilled advocates will refer you to an attorney if need be and will also teach you how to be an effective advocate for your child, should you be unable to find a professional.

The majority of professional advocates will also consider their role to include the facilitation of a collaborative and positive relationship with school districts and school to the fullest possible extent while simultaneously holding them accountable to the state and federal laws that have been put in place to protect your child. Advocates work tirelessly to maintain a respectful, professional, and collaborative atmosphere in meetings, to encourage the whole team to remain focused on the educational needs of your child. This is, at times, the most challenging and important role that they must fulfill.

CHOOSING THE RIGHT ONE

After you have made the decision that you need the assistance of an autism advocate, you're going to be faced with the dilemma of figuring out which one to choose. While I will answer some questions that will provide you with essential information, it is imperative that you feel a connection with the advocate you eventually select. You must have confidence in them and trust them as well. You will generally be able to tell whether they are a good match from your first exchange.

One of the first questions you should be asking an advocate is what their training and education is. Currently, there is no training required to become an advocate. However, Massachusetts, as well as several other states, have participated in a pilot study of a nationally-designed curriculum. There is likely to be a more formal standard for people wanting to become advocates at some point in the future. Until this happens, Massachusettsans - that is, people living in Massachusetts - have the luxury of the Parent Consultant Training Institutes, which are provided by the Federation for Children with Special Needs. Thanks to this thorough training series, many advocates receive preliminary exposure to the field and begin to develop their skills. Sadly, the program is unique to Massachusetts and does not exist in many other states.

Next, you should be asking your advocate what they do to keep updated. Most advocates, or good ones, at least, will continually build upon their skills by attending seminars and workshops. Changes are continuously being made to the way that special education laws are implemented and interpreted, which is why it is so important for advocates to keep themselves up-to-date. In this regard, the Special Needs Advocacy Network is a helpful non-profit professional organization that offers training, workshops, and professional information related to special education. If your advocate cites SPaN, then they're very likely worth their salt. The organization is also a useful tool for parents that are looking to become their child's advocates, a topic we'll discuss later in the chapter.

You should also inquire about the duration that your advocate has been advocating at a professional level. Most advocates will agree that, while initial and ongoing training is important, working in the field is the best way to get the hang of advocating. Advocates, through experience, find and develop the style that works best for both them and their clients, and practical experience can also help them expand their resource network so that they can easily find the help that your child needs. Whatever the experience level may be, you should feel that your advocate is being open and honest about it and clear about whether their particular experience will suit your needs. You're certainly going to want an advocate that has plenty of experience with your specific needs - timelines are often short, and the consequences of error are much too serious for anything less.

Find out whether or not your advocate has worked for other families in your child's school district before. While it's not vital, it is generally useful for an advocate to have experience in your district. This is because, by working in a school district, they get a firsthand experience of the programs that that district offers, an idea of how the district operates, and get to work with the staff. If an advocate is working on a particularly challenging case in your district, they may refer you to another advocate to avoid the chance that their involvement with the challenging case will bias the district against yours.

Due to these situations, having an advocate that has not had much experience with your district can sometimes be advantageous. If you are thinking of hiring an advocate with no experience with your district, be sure to ask them how important they think experience is for your specific situation, and the steps they would take if they felt they needed more information about that district.

Will your advocate have enough time to take on your case? You should be thorough when outlining your needs to your advocate, as most will handle numerous cases at once, and try to monitor their workload as closely as possible. During your first discussion with your advocate, your needs, and the estimated number of hours it will take to achieve your objectives, will be made clearer, and if your needs surpass that of which the advocate can accommodate, you should ask them to refer you to another advocate.

Finally, and this is perhaps the most important point, you should ask your advocate how much they charge and what exactly they charge for. You should be sure to get this information when interviewing prospective candidates - most advocates will present their fee structure when you first meet with them. Additionally, the majority of advocates will provide you with a fee agreement that details the fee structure and any other limitations or policies that they feel you should be aware of. Rates will vary, as will the services that are billed.

Nearly all advocates will charge a rate based on hours, and most will, in some way, charge for a travel time. Find out what your advocate will consider billable activities, and it is also within reason to inquire about an estimated number of hours involved in your particular case, at least in its initial stage. Note that some advocates will request a retainer or deposit upfront, while others may prefer to charge you for hours as they are worked.

The styles of advocates will vary, just as the styles of parents do. Once you have identified a few qualified candidates that you believe could help your child, decide on one that is compatible with both your personality and objectives. Speaking to them should feel comfortable and natural, and you should not be afraid to share important information about your child with them. You are about to embark on a journey of mutually understood goals and objectives.

ADVOCATING FOR YOUR CHILD WHEN NO ONE ELSE CAN

You may find yourself in a situation where you've searched and searched for the right professional advocate to suit your needs but can't seem to find one that is compatible. In this case, you may need to act as your child's advocate, which can be a daunting task, especially if you have no experience as an autism advocate.

As a parent of a child with autism, you have two main goals: to build a healthy working relationship with your child's school and to ensure that their school is providing your child with a free appropriate public education that includes specially designed instruction to meet the unique needs of your child. What are your long-term goals for your child? What do you picture for them in the future? If you are like most parents, then you are probably focused on the present and have not given the future much thought.

Do you expect your child to be a self-sufficient, independent member of the community and society? While some children with autism will need some level of assistance as adults, most will grow up to become adults that get married, hold jobs, and live independently. If you start with a vision of what you want your child to achieve in the future, then you will already be more likely to achieve your goals as your child's advocate. Accepting a role in leadership as your child's autism advocate will bolster your position in encounters with teachers, doctors, therapists, caregivers, and all others who offer services to your child. Keep in mind that you are on a steep learning curve and will not be able to change things overnight, but if you persist and do your best, you will, in time, be able to make a meaningful difference.

To become an expert on autism, you don't need a fancy degree - you are already an expert on your child. However, if you want people to take you seriously as an advocate, you will need to know everything from the preliminary diagnosis to treatment options, state and federal laws protecting those with disabilities, and educational choices. You'll need to learn the abbreviations and jargon associated with autism.

Critical thinking is another invaluable skill that you will need as an autism advocate since, when researching autism, you will be exposed to endless streams of information from blogs, online articles, magazines, newspapers, and books such as this one. You will need to constantly weigh what to do for your child and what to believe. It is important to think for yourself - examine the evidence, benefits, and detriments, and take note of how your emotions are influencing your thinking.

Being proactive and the ability to speak with authority are two skills that I cannot emphasize enough. Even if you have never been a powerful speaker, you can learn and practice discussing autism with authority in medical appointments, school meetings, and other settings. You have to remember that you are the only living authority on your child and are the best person alive to frame their situation in the most compassionate way possible. Even if you don't think of yourself as a courageous person, you can become a powerful and outspoken advocate when it comes to the best interests of your child.

Preparation is key as well. Having your documents organized at all times, from the initial diagnosis of your child to their numerous evaluations each year, will make your life much simpler and empower you further as an advocate. I recommend keeping a file of all of the important documents and paperwork, as well as taking notes during meetings and phone calls requesting insurance coverage or other services. You should also think about keeping a journal for you and your child to record their strengths, experiences, and challenges, as well as artwork and the like, so that you can share it with new babysitters, teachers, and even relatives to give them some insight into your child's life.

As your child's advocate, you should be collaborating and focusing on being a team builder, constantly working toward synergy and working together to pool your human resources and help your child. Your team could include a specialty physician that regularly meets your child and the aide to your child's special education, who sees them at school daily. Even if your daily experiences leave you feeling stressed and exhausted, you should always try to have quality interactions and focus on the long-term. If you're an amicable teammate, you'll be presented with plenty of advantages.

Chapter References

LeBlanc, S., & Riley, C. (n.d.). *Basic Guidelines for Choosing an Advocate for Your Child*. Asperger / Autism Network. Retrieved February 12, 2021, from https://www.aane.org/basic-guidelines-choosing-advocate-child/

Wright, P. W. D. (n.d.). *How to become an advocate for your child | Autism Support Network*. Autism Support Network. Retrieved February 12, 2021, from http://www.autismsupportnetwork.com/news/how-become-advocate-your-child-autism-302201945

Davis, M. K. S. (2018, October 12). *Advocates: Qualities to Look for and Choosing the Correct One for YOU*. Indiana Resource Center for Autism. https://www.iidc.indiana.edu/irca/articles/advocates-qualities-to-look-for-and-choosing-the-correct-one-for-you.html

Dower, E. (2020, December 29). 7 Ways to Be an Everyday Advocate for Your Child with Autism. FamilyEducation. https://www. familyeducation.com/life/coping-autism/7-ways-be-everyday-advocate-your-child-autism?slide=5#fen-gallery

FINAL WORDS

Autism is not an easy condition to deal with, both for you as a parent and for your child who is on the spectrum. It presents a plethora of challenges each and every day, from communication and bonding to aggression, frustration, and much more. Being the parent of a child with autism is not an easy task, and it requires far more effort from you than being a parent of neurotypical children. However, no matter how many challenges and frustrations your child may present, you still love them more than anything and want the best for them at all times.

Raising a child with ASD does not have to be difficult, and if you are willing to put the effort in, it can actually be a beautiful experience. Children and adults with ASD have a lot to teach us, both about themselves and about ourselves, and it is essential that you are willing to learn from your child just as much as you are willing to help and teach them. There is something extra-special about each and every child on the spectrum, and giving them all of the special attention and care that they need will be the secret to unlocking their potential.

If there is one thing that I hope you learned from this book, it is that you are not alone, and there are so many parents out there that share your experiences. Being the parent of a child with autism can often feel lonely, especially if you don't feel like you have a support system that you can lean on when you become overwhelmed with stress, frustration, and dejection. I hope that you loved reading this book and that you will be able to learn all there is to know about your child!

Chapter references

Applied Behavioral Analysis. (2017, November 30). *5 Tips for Talking to Neurotypical Kids About Siblings with ASD*. Applied Behavioral Analysis | How to Become an Applied Behavior Analyst. https://www.appliedbehavioranalysisedu.org/5-tips-for-talking-to-neurotypical-kids-about-siblings-with-asd/

AR Organization for Autism Research. (n.d.). *Brothers, sisters, and autism: a parent's guide to supporting autistic siblings*. Retrieved February 24, 2021, from https://researchautism.org/wp-content/uploads/2016/04/OAR_SiblingResource_Parents_2015.pdf

Autism Parenting Magazine. (2020, August 8). *Simple Ways You Can Help Strengthen the ASD Sibling Relationship*. https://www.autismparentingmagazine.com/strengthening-asd-sibling-relationship/

Autism Speaks. (n.d.). *Sibling's Guide to Autism*. Retrieved February 24, 2021, from https://www.autismspeaks.org/sites/default/files/2018-08/Siblings%20Guide%20to%20Autism.pdf

Family Life With Autism. (n.d.). UniversalClass.Com. Retrieved February 24, 2021, from https://www.universalclass.com/articles/special-education/family-life-with-autism.htm

Promoting Positive Sibling Relationships. (n.d.). Marcus Autism Center. Retrieved February 24, 2021, from https://www.marcus.org/autism-resources/autism-tips-and-resources/promoting-positive-sibling-relationships

Rudy, L. J. (2019, December 4). *10 Activities to Enjoy With Your Autistic Child*. Verywell Health. https://www.verywellhealth.com/hobbies-activities-autistic-child-260365

Siblings. (2014, April 16). Autism Society. https://www.autism-society.org/living-with-autism/autism-and-your-family/siblings/

Siblings of autistic children: experiences, relationships and support. (2020, December 10). Raising Children Network. https://raisingchildren.net.au/autism/communicating-relationships/family-relationships/siblings-asd

Wheeler, M. M. (n.d.). *Siblings Perspectives: Some Guidelines for Parents*. Indiana Resource Center for Autism. Retrieved February 24, 2021, from https://www.iidc.indiana.edu/irca/articles/siblings-perspectives-some-guidelines-for-parents.html